Dictionary of Pharmacognosy

Dictionary of Pharmacognosy

Sanskriti Sharma

IVY Publishing House
Delhi—110 095

Published by
IVY Publishing House
Delhi-110095
Sole Distributors
Sarup & Sons
4740/23, Ansari Road
Darya Ganj, New Delhi-110002
Ph.: 011-23281029, 23244664, 41010989
Fax: 011-23277098
email-sarupandsonsin@hotmail.com

Dictionary of Pharmacognosy

ISBN 81-7890-154-4
1st Edition 2007

Printed in India

Laser Typesetting at Jain Computers and Printed at Roshan Offset Press, Delhi.

Preface

This dictionary of Pharmacognosy is essentially compilation of terms related to various aspects of Pharmacognosy. The selection of terms included in this dictionary has been carried out in such a way that this dictionary explores the importance of Pharmacognosy. The terms have been arranged in alphabetical order. The technical language used for explaining terms is simple and easy to understand. This dictionary is suitable for diploma, undergraduate and postgraduate students of Pharmacy.

A

Acclimatization

The biological process whereby an organism adapts to a new environment. One example is the process of developing microorganisms that degrade toxic wastes in the environment.

Accommodation Schedule

Defines all areas that can influence unit operations required for manufacturing, and relationships and flows between them.

Account Policy

Specifies how passwords must be defined and employed for all user accounts on a system. It specifically addresses the issues of password aging, password uniqueness, and locking a user account because of invalid logon attempts. CFR 21 Part 11 mandates technical controls in these areas specifically.

Acetyl CoA, Acetyl Coenzyme A

Condensation product of coenzyme A and acetic acid.

Acetylcholine

Ester of choline and acetic acid, widespread in the body; functions as a neurotransmitter at synapses and neuromuscular junctions.

Acid

A compound of an electronegative element or radical with

hydrogen; it form salts by replacing all or part of the hydrogen with an electropositive element or radical. Or, a hydrogen-containing substance that when dissolved in water dissociates to produce one or more hydrogen ions (H+).

Acid Feed

Injection of an acid into a liquid stream to make it less alkaline (pH adjustment).

Aconite

It is the dried roots of *Aconitum napellus* Linn.

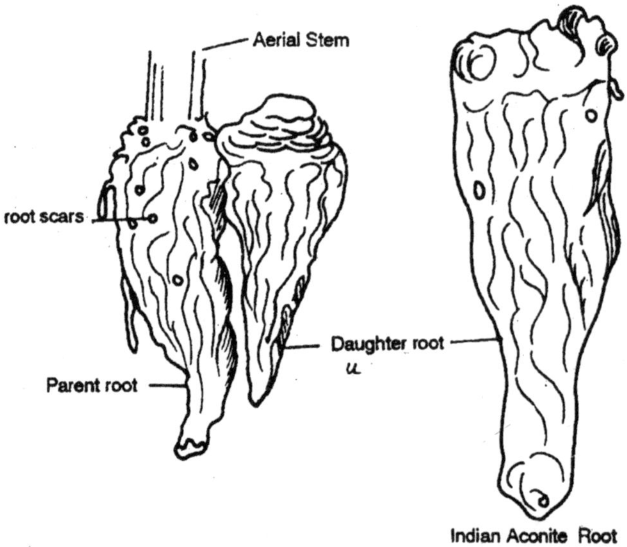

Aconite

Action Point

A value set to identify when a parameter has drifted outside the operating range (Acceptance Criteria). A documented response is usually required.

Activated Carbon

Material used to adsorb organic impurities from water. Derived from wood, lignite, pulp-mill char, blood, etc. The source material is initially charred at high temperature to convert it to carbon. The carbon is then "activated" by oxidation from exposure to high temperature steam. It comes in granular or powdered form.

Active Immunity

The formation of an antibody that can be stimulated by infection or vaccination.

Active Ingredient

Any component that is intended to furnish pharmacological activity or other direct effect in the diagnosis, cure, mitigation, treatment, or prevention of disease, or to affect the structure or any function of the body of man or other animals. The term includes those components that may undergo chemical change in the manufacture of the drug product and are present in the drug product in a modified form intended to furnish the specified activity or effect.

Active ingredient/constituent

One or more molecules which have been isolated from the plant matrix and scientifically established to have a specific physiological activity, both in isolation and within the context of the whole herb or extract. This concept comes from conventional pharmacy where an 'active ingredient' might be part of a solution containing a number of other ingredients including carriers or 'excipients.' Active ingredients generally exhibit a 'dose-dependent response' - in other words, the more one takes, the more activity one gets. Many herbalists think that the entire herb or extract is really the 'active ingredient/s' in which many constituents are acting together - synergistically.

Active Site

The region of a protein molecule that binds the specific substrate and chemically modifies it into the new product (in an enzyme) or interacts with it (in a receptor).

Active Transport

Energy-requiring transport of a solution across a membrane in the direction of increasing concentration.

Acute Toxicity

Adverse effects resulting from a single exposure or dose of a chemical; immediate effect.

Actual Yield

The quantity that is actually produced at any appropriate phase of manufacture, processing, or packaging of a particular drug product.

Acupuncture

Techniques for treating some painful conditions and for regional anaesthesia by passing long thin needles through the skin to specific points.

Adaptogen

A substance that increases resistance to stress and balances and normalises body functions.

Adenine (A)

A purine base, 6-aminopurine, occurring in RNA (ribonucleic acid) and DNA (deoxyribonucleic acid) and as a component of adenosine triphosphate.

Adsorption

Adhesion of the molecules of a gas, liquid or dissolved substance to a surface because of chemical or electrical attraction - typically accomplished with granular activated carbon to remove dissolved organics and chlorine. The attachment of charged particles to the chemically active groups on the surface and in the pores of an ion exchanger.

Adventitious Agents

Acquired, sporadic, accidental contaminants.

Adverse Agents
Undesired effects or toxicity due to exposure (often but not limited to a drug or medical device).

Adverse Drug Reaction (ADR)
An undesirable effect that may be caused by a study drug.

Advisory Alarm
An alarm indicating a drift of a monitored parameter toward an out-of-spec condition. It is advisory in that no GMP violation has occurred, and is used to advise corrective action before an action alarm can happen.

Aerobe
An organism that can live and grow only in the presence of oxygen.
1. Facultative aerobe: one which normally thrives in the absence of oxygen, but which may acquire the faculty of living in the presence of oxygen.
2. Obligate aerobe: one that cannot live without air.

Aerobia
The plural of aerobe.

Aerobic
Living in air.

Aerobic Bacteria
Bacteria capable of growing in the presence of Oxygen.

Aerobion
see: Aerobe

Aerosol
A product that is dispensed by a propellant from a metal can up to a maximum size of 33.8 fluid ounces (1000 mL) or a glass or plastic bottle up to a size of 4 fluid ounces (118.3 mL), other than a rim-vented container.

Aerosol

A gaseous suspension of fine (100μm or smaller in size) solid or liquid particles.

Aerosol Photometer

Light-scattering mass concentration indicating instrument with a threshold sensitivity of at least 10 to the negative third power microgram per liter for 0.3μm diameter DOP (Dioctyl Phthalate) concentrations over a range of 10 to the fifth power times the threshold sensitivity. Photometers may include hand-held remote meter probes that can scan for airborne contaminants in HEPA filters, in penetrations around frames, seals and plenums, and in hoods and work stations.

AES

see: Auger Electron Spectroscopy

Agar

A complex mixture of polysaccharides obtained from marine red algae, used as an emulsion stabilizer in foods, as a sizing in fabrics, as a gelling agent and as a solid substrate or media for the laboratory culture of microorganisms. Agar melts at 100°C and when cooled below 44°C forms a stiff and transparent gel. Microorganisms are seeded and grown on the surface of the gel.

Agarose

A highly purified form of agar.

Agarose Gel Electrophoresis

A method used to separate, identify, and purify molecules of different molecular weight and/or structure. It is specifically applied to the separation of protein or DNA fragments where it is rapid, simple, and accurate, and the separated molecules can be visualized directly by staining with dyes. The electrophoretic migration rate of molecules through agarose gel is dependent on the following parameters:

1. Molecular size: molecules pass through the gel at rates that are inversely proportional to the log of their molecular weight.
2. Agarose concentration: a molecule of a given size migrates

at different rates through gels containing different concentrations of agarose.
3. Molecular conformation: a molecule of the same molecular weight but of a different conformation will migrate at different rates. Generally, closed circular or globular forms will migrate faster than linear forms.
4. Electric current: at low voltages the rate of migration is proportional to the voltage, but as the voltage is increased the rate of migration of high molecular weight fragments is increased differentially.

Agene

Nitrogen Trichloride (NCl3).

Agglomerate

Suspended solids clustered together to form larger clumps or masses that are easier to remove by filtration or settling.

Agglutination

The sticking together of insoluble antigens such as bacteria, viruses or erythrocytes by a particular antibody. Agglutination assays are used to type human blood before a transfusion.

Aglycone

Some molecules (such as anthocyanidins or isoflavones) can exist with or without a sugar group attached to them. When they are without the sugar group, they are known as aglycones ('a-' means 'without'). When they have the sugar group, they are known as glycosides.

AHF (Antihemophilic Factor)

In the clotting of blood it is also known as Factor VIII.

Airborne Particulate Cleanliness Classes

Statistically allowable number of particles equal to, or larger than 0.5µm in size per cubic foot of air. According to ISO 14644-1, a classification number, N, shall designate airborne particulate cleanliness.

Air Change Rate

The number of times the total air volume of a defined space is replaced in a given unit of time. This is computed by dividing the total volume of the subject space (in cubic feet) into the total volume of air exhausted from (or supplied to) the space per unit of time.

Air Cleaners

Filtration systems that may be freestanding or installed in a ceiling or wall to remove contaminants such as bacteria, viruses, and dust from the air. Air cleaners may incorporate HEPA filters.

Airflow Visualization

Using chemical smoke or fog to visualize flow patterns in a cleanroom or clean space.

Air-Lift Bioreactor

A reactor in which the source of agitation is air sparged upwards through a draft tube - most widely used for cell culture applications and monoclonal antibody production.

Airlock

A room or space designed to act as a means of segregating areas of different air classification or quality. It may contain a method to remove particulate contamination from clean room garments as personnel pass through, and usually includes HEPA filtered air supply and interlocking doors. Airlocks pressure will "float" between those of the spaces being protected. With all doors closed, the airlock pressure will be somewhere between that of the highest adjoining room and that of the lowest adjoining room as air flows through it from room to room. "Ventilated airlocks" are in neutral ducted air balance (supply CFM = return CFM).

Air Velocity Meters/Monitors

Meters to measure and indicate the force and speed of airflow. Meters may use a variety of probes for measuring near HEPA filters and at right angles. Monitors check and record air velocity.

Ajwain

Ajwain (also known as **Carom, Ajowan, Bishop's Weed** and **Seeds Of Bishop's Weed**), is an uncommon spice except in certain areas of Asia. It is the small seed-like fruit of the Bishop's Weed plant, *(Trachyspermum ammi syn. Carum copticum)*, egg-shaped and grayish in colour. The plant has a similarity to parsley.

Ajwain is often confused with lovage seed; even some dictionaries mistakenly state that ajwain comes from the lovage plant.

Raw ajwain smells almost exactly like thyme because it also contains thymol, but is more aromatic and less subtle in taste, as well as slightly bitter and pungent. Even a small amount of raw ajwain will completely dominate the flavor of a dish. In Indian cuisine, ajwain is almost never used raw, but either dry-roasted or fried in ghee. This develops a much more subtle and complex aroma, somewhat similar to caraway but "brighter".

Ajwain originated in the Middle East, possibly in Egypt. It is now primarily grown and used in the Indian Subcontinent, but also in Iran, Egypt and Afghanistan. It is sometimes used as an ingredient in berebere, an Ethiopian spice mixture.

The dried fruits of the plant are used. Because they look like seeds, some call Ajwain, **Ajwain seed**. The flavour of this spice can be improved by roasting the small fruits in a dry pan.

It is used in India and Africa, and one of the most common uses is with lentils. Supposedly it can reduce the gassy effect of beans when the two are cooked together. One suggestion is to use it along with cumin, whenever cumin is called for.

Alarms

Audible or visual signals used to warn of unacceptable conditions at monitored sites. They may be buzzers, horns, speakers, bells, or warning lights. They can be Advisory, Alert, or Action alarms. The first two are for operation and maintenance information, to alert of abnormal situations that do not compromise product SISPQ. The Action alarm is for GMP records, indicating that product SISPQ may have been compromised, but Alert alarms are also usually recorded.

Albumin

Commonly, the white of egg is a simple protein widely distributed throughout the tissues and fluid of plants and animals. Soluble in pure water it is also precipitable from a solution by mineral acids, and coagulable by heat in acid or neutral solution.

Albuminoid

Resembling albumin, a simple protein present in horny and cartilaginous tissues, insoluble in neutral solvents. Keratin, elastin, and collagen are albuminoids.

Alert Point

Used in determining when a parameter is drifting toward extremes of the operating range.

Alfalfa (Medicago sativa)

A blood purifier; reduces and prevents symptoms caused by arthritis, bursitis, and gout9; lowers cholesterol10. Contains natural fluorides ,preventing tooth decay and helps rebuild decaying teeth. Alfalfa contains eight essential digestive enzymes and eight essential amino acids of protein and a high chlorophyll content. Extremely rich source of Beta-Carotene, Minerals, Trace elements, and vitamins A,B-1, B-6, B-12, C, D, E, K, Biotin, Folic Acid, Niacin and Pantothenic Acid. Mineras are Calcium, copper, Iron, Magnesium, Phosphorus, Potassium and Zinc.

Aliquot

Of, pertaining to, or designating an exact divisor or factor of a quantity, specially of an integer. To divide out a sample to multiple containers for multiple analytical tests.

Alkaloids

Alkaloids are arguably the most potent therapeutic compounds and have been manufactured as various allopathic drugs, including the pain-killer morphine and the anti-malarial quinine. Derived from amino acids, alkaloids represent a varied and complex class of nitrogenous crystalline or oily compounds. Alkaloid levels in a given botanical change in the course of the day and are not homogeneous, which makes them difficult to define (Tyler et al., 186). Their presence appears to be most prevalent in the Fabaceae/Leguminosae, Papaveraceae, Ranunculaceae, Rubiaceae, Solanaceae, and Berberidacea families. Plant genera providing the highest yield of alkaloids are Nicotiana, Vinca, Strychnos, Papaver sominifera, and Rauwolfia serpentia.

Pyrrolidine, tropane, or solanaceous alkaloids effect the peripheral nervous system, inhibiting the parasympathetic nervous system and stimulating the sympathetic. Pupils dilate, secretions slow, and the vagus nerve is inhibited (causing vasodilation, bronchial dilation, and reduced peristalsis).

Pyridine and piperidine alkaloids represent a class which affects the central nervous system, reduces appetite, and contains other properties usually diuretic or diaphoretic in action. Nicotine, lobeline, and coniine are examples. Coniine is extremely toxic.

Pyrrolizidine alkaloids are under fire today as chemists and doctors try to determine the human hepatotoxicity of these agents which can damage liver veins, causing hepatic veno-occlusive disease. Toxicity to livestock is demonstrated by the fact that 50% of livestock deaths occur through the ingestion of a plant that contains these alkaloids. Because of five well-publicized deaths (one of which was the teratogenic poisoning of a fetus) following the consumption of an herb(comfrey) that had been regarded as safe, plant families in which pyrrolizidine alkaloids are most often found (Boraginacea, Asteraceae/Compositae, and Fabaceae/Leguminosae) are of immense concern to both herbalists and the FDA.

Indole alkaloids are derived from tryptophan, and apart from the few with hallucinogenic effects, indoles such as serotonin, harmine and reserpine have a sedative effect on the central nervous system. Other constituents in this category are cytostatic, antileukemic, or are able to act on the ratio of oxygen and glucose to the cell, specifically increasing oxygen to deprived areas.

Quinoline alkaloids are named from quinoline in the cinchona plant, and refers to the quinoline alkaloids developed in the nucleus from tryptophan. Included in this group are quinine, the anti-malaria medication, and quinidine, which calms the

heart in tachycardiasis and arrhythmia, and others. Chinchonine is an astringent and a bitter. Isoquinoline alkaloids are derived from tyrosine and phenylalanine.
The therapeutic value of this class of alkaloid differs according to the sub-categories, which include simple, benzyl, Papaveraceae, codeine, protopine, protoberberine, and ipecac isoquinolines. The protoberberines, which include berberine, hydrastine, and canadine, are anti-bacterial, anti-protozoal, astringent, tonic, bitter tasting, and respiratory, vasomotor, and circulatory stimulants.
2. Natural occurring nitrogen containing compounds usually having heterocyclic structures and displaying pharmacological activity. Alkaloids are usually classed according to the chemical structure of their main nucleus, e.g. indole alkaloids, isoquinoline, alkaloids, etc.

Alkalinity

An expression of the total amount of basic anions (hydroxyl groups) present in a solution. In water analysis, it also represents the presence of carbonate, bicarbonate, and occasionally borate, silicate, and phosphate salts that react to produce hydroxyl groups. Bicarbonate and carbonate ions are expected to be in most waters. Hydroxide may occur in water that has been softened by the lime soda process or has been in contact with fresh concrete. Alkalinity furnishes a guide in choosing appropriate treatment of either raw water or plant effluents.

Allantoic Fluid

The clear white portion of an egg. In influenza vaccine manufacturing, the virus is propagated in the embryonic chick and sloughed into the allantoic fluid that is harvested to produce the vaccine.

Allele

Alternative form of a genetic locus; a single allele for each locus is inherited separately from each parent (e.g., at a locus for eye color the allele might result in blue or brown eyes)

Allergenic Extract

An extract in a solvent of a substance that causes an allergic reaction. They are relative crude drugs by contemporary standards and are manufactured by specialty companies and in some cases, by a practicing allergist. Also, allergenic extracts are generally difficult to filter since they most frequently are extracts of natural substances such as foods, house dust, animal hair, etc.

Allyl group

A functional group composed of $H_2C{=}CH{-}CH_2{-}R$, found in many of the sulfur compounds of Garlic as well as in other organic molecules; this group was actually named after the Latin for Garlic, Allium, by a chemist researching Garlic oil in the 1840s.

Alpha-adrenergic receptors

A site in the autonomic nervous system where excitatory responses occur when adrenergic agents such as norepinephrine and epinephrine are released.

Alum

Aluminum sulfate, commonly added during municipal water treatment to cause insoluble colloids to coalesce into larger particles that can be removed by settling.

Alzheimer's Disease

A disease that causes memory loss, personality changes, dementia and, ultimately, death. Not all cases are inherited, but genes have been found for familial forms of Alzheimer's disease.

Ambient

The normal environment conditions such as temperature, relative humidity, or room pressure of a particular area under consideration.

Amchur

Amchur is dried mango used as spices in south and southeast Asia.

Amine

A substance that may be derived from ammonia by the replacement of one or more of the hydrogen atoms by hydrocarbon radicals.

Amino Acids

Any of a group of twenty hydrocarbon molecules (containing the radical group NH2) linked together in various combinations to form proteins in living things. Synthesized by living cells or obtained as essential components of the diet of human and animals, these twenty amino acids are divided into four (4) groups on the basis of their side-chain properties:

1. Neutral, hydrophobic side chains,
2. Neutral, hydrophilic side chains,
3. Acid, hydrophilic side chains,
4. Basic, hydrophilic side chains.

In addition to the twenty common amino acids there are less common derivatives (e.g. hydroxyproline, found in collagen) formed by the modification of a common amino acid.

An organic compound with an amine group ($-NH_2$), a carboxylic acid group (-COOH), a hydrogen atom, and a varying 'R' group bonded to the central carbon atom (the 'alpha' carbon). There are 21 'standard' amino acids from which proteins are composed, and many additional modified types. Alliin, from Garlic, is an example of a modified amino acid.

Amla

The drug consists of the fresh or dried fruit of *Emblica officinalis* L or *phyllanthus embelica* Linn.

Amla

Amino Acids

In plants, amino acids are broken down into two groups, protein, and non-protein. There are twenty amino acids, derived from the acid hydrolysates of plant proteins (as with animal proteins). Plant proteins are essential for carrying out specific cellular functions both internally and externally. Plant proteins are seed-based store-houses for nitrogen and guard against would-be predators. Some are toxic to humans, some are of daily necessity in the human diet. Some, furthermore, have been developed into specific drugs: L-Dopa, from fava beans and other Fabaceae/Leguminosae, is used in the treatment of Parkinson's disease; L-Cysteine, found in all plants, is used in eye drops and topical antibiotics. L-Arganine stimulates the pituitary gland to release growth hormone. L-Aspartic acid is present in coffee, liquorice, sugar cane, sugar beet, and is neuro-excitatory. It is the phytochemical responsible for so-called 'sugar highs,' and is in aspartame.

Ampholyte

Amphoteric electrolyte. Electrolyte that can either give up or take on a hydrogen ion and can thus behave as either an acid or a base.

Amphoteric

Having two opposite characteristics.

Ampicillin

An antibiotic widely used in clinical treatment and rDNA research. It is a derivative of penicillin, which kills bacteria by interfering with the synthesis of the cell wall.

Amplification

An increase in the number of copies of a specific DNA fragment; can be In Vivo or In Vitro.

Amplification

The production of additional copies of a chromosomal sequence, found as either intrachromosomal or extrachromosomal DNA.

Ampoule or Ampule

A small glass vial sealed after filling and one of the earliest devices developed for safe storage of sterile injectable unit.

Amyotrophic Lateral Sclerosis

An inherited, fatal degenerative nerve disorder, also known as Lou Gehrig's disease.

Anabolism

The constructive phase of metabolism whereby nutrient substances are utilised for the repair and growth of the organisms. Opposite of catabolism.
2. The intracellular process involved in the synthesis of more complex compounds than those involved in catabolism (for example, glucose to glycogen) and requires energy.

Anaerobe

A microorganism that thrives best, or only, when deprived of oxygen.
1. Facultative anaerobe: one able to grow in the presence or absence of free oxygen.
2. Obligate or obligatory anaerobe: one that will grow only in the absence of free oxygen.

Anaerobic

Relating to an anaerobe.

Anaerobic Bacteria

Bacteria capable of growing in the absence of Oxygen.

Analog

Pertaining to data that consists of continuously variable physical qualities.

Analytical Data Interchange (ANDI)

A generic file format. It was common practice before CFR 21 Part 11 to save information from analytical instruments in this file format. The disadvantage now is that the approach does not allow replaying of data on a different system to yield the same result.

Analytical Method

Small scale process used to characterize and/or separate a mixture, a compound, or an unknown material into its constituent parts or elements.

Ancillary Material

Material used in preparing drugs that does not become a component of the drug (e.g. steam, air, N2, DI water).

Anecdotal

Hearsay evidence presented to support a scientific hypothesis.

Anemometer

A device that measures air speed.

Angelica

Angelica is a genus of the Umbilliferous family Apiaceae, with about 50 species of tall perennial herbs 1-2 m tall with large bipinnate leaves and large compound umbels of white or greenish-white flowers. Some members are grown as a flavoring agent and for their medicinal properties. The most notable of these is Garden Angelica (Angelica archangelica) which is commonly known just as Angelica. Cystalised strips of angelica stem are green in colour and are sold as decorative and flavoursome cake decoration material.

Sea watch or Seacoast Angelica, Angelica lucida, has been eaten as a sort of "wild celery".

Helps regulate menstruation, diaphoretic11; diuretic; expectorant for coughs, bronchitis and pleurisy, particularly when symptoms are accompanied by fever, colds, or influenza; relieves gas, can help stimulate appetite; helps the skin eliminate toxins; may be used in anorexia nervosa.

Angiotensin converting enzyme (ACE)

A hydrolase responsible for the conversion of angiotensin I to the vasoactive angiotensin II. Drugs that inhibit ACE are used to treat hypertension and congestive heart failure.

Angstrom (?)

A unit of length equal to one hundred-millionth of a centimeter (one ten-thousandth of a micron) used especially to specify radiation wavelengths.

Anneal

The process by which the complementary base pairs in DNA strands combine.

Annealing

A treatment process for steel in which the metal is heated and held at a suitable temperature and then cooled at a suitable rate for the purpose of reducing hardness, improving machinability, facilitating cold working, producing a desired microstructure, or obtaining desired mechanical, physical, or other properties.

Anion

A negatively charged particle or ion.

Anion Exchange Resin

An ion exchange material that removes anions from solution by exchanging them with hydroxyl ions.

Anise

Anise (stressed on the first syllable, rhyming with "Janice"), or more rarely **anís** (stressed on the second syllable, as "a niece") (Pimpinella anisum) is an herb in the family Apiaceae (formerly Umbelliferae) whose seed-like fruit (also called aniseed) is used in sweet baking as well as in anise-flavored liqueurs (e.g. Ouzo). The fruit consists of two united carpels, called a cremocarp, and has a strong aromatic taste and a powerful odour. Anise seed is also used in some curries and seafood dishes, and is used as a breath sweetener and digestive aid.

All above-ground parts of the young anise plant are also eaten as a vegetable. The stems resemble those of celery in texture and are much milder in flavor than the fruits. Anise is believed to be a galactagogue.

By distillation the fruit yields the volatile oil of anise, which is useful in the treatment of flatulence and colic in children. It may be given as Aqua Anisi, in doses of one or more ounces, or as the Spiritus Anisi, in doses of 5-20 minims.

The primary constituent of the oil (up to 90%) is anethole, $C_{10}H_{12}O$ or $C_6H_4[1.4](OCH_3)(CH:CH.CH_3.)$ It also contains methyl chavicol, anisic aldehyde, anisic acid, and a terpene. The Chinese star anise also contains anethole but is botanically unrelated to anise. Because of its similar taste and aroma, it has recently come into use in the West as a (cheaper) substitute for anise in baking as well as in liquor production. According to Easton's Bible Dictionary (1897), the term anise in the Christian (Matt. 23:23) refers to the herb known today as dill (Anethum' or Peucedanum graveolens).

Annatto

Annatto is a derivative of the seed of the achiote trees (Bixa orellana L.) of tropical regions of the Americas, used to produce a red food coloring. It is used in cheese, margarine, butter, rice and smoked fish. Annatto is commonly found in Latin America and Caribbean cuisines as both a coloring agent and for flavoring. Central and South American Indians used the seeds to make a body paint, and as a lipstick. For this reason, the achiote is sometimes called the lipstick-tree."

Antibiotic

A chemical substance, produced by a microorganism, which has the capacity, in low concentrations, to inhibit or even destroy bacteria and other microorganisms. The definition may be expanded to include higher plants as a source.

2. An organic substance of microbial origin (usually mold or actinomycete bacteria) that is either toxic or growth inhibiting for other organisms. Also with the advent of synthetic methods of production, a substance produced by a microorganism or a similar substance (produced wholly or partly by chemical synthesis) which, in low concentrations, inhibits the growth of other microorganisms. Penicillin, tetracycline, and erythromycin are examples of antibiotics.

Antibody

Complex glycoproteins produced by B-lymphocytes in the presence of an antigen. Antibodies, all of which are immunoglobulins can combine with specific antigens to destroy or control them, providing protection against most common infections.

2. A modified protein molecule present in the blood serum or plasma (and other body fluids), whose activity is associated chiefly with gamma globulin. Produced by the immune system in response to exposure to a foreign substance, it is the body's protective mechanism against infection and disease. An antibody is characterized by a structure complementary to the foreign substance, the antigen that provokes its formation, and is thus capable of binding specifically to the foreign substance to neutralize it.

Antigen

A protein marker on the surface of cells that identifies the cell as "self" or "non-self"; antigens stimulate production of antibodies by B-lymphocytes which can neutralise or destroy the antigen bearing cell, and also can stimulate cytotoxic responses by granulocytes, monocytes, and lymphocytes.

2. Any of various foreign substances such as bacteria, viruses, endotoxins, exotoxins, foreign proteins, pollen, and vaccines, whose entry into an organism induces an immune response (antibody production, lymphokine production, or both) directed specifically against that molecule. Response may be demonstrated as an increased reaction, such as hypersensitivity (usually protein or a complex of protein and polysaccharide, or occasionally a polysaccharide of high molecular weight), a circulating antibody that reacts with the antigen, or some degree of immunity to infectious disease if the antigen was a microorganism or its products.

Antioxidant

A substance which protects tissues from damage by stabilizing harmful free radicals. Free radicals have an unpaired electron, which is very reactive; antioxidants donate a companion electron to the free radical to 'calm it down' so that it doesn't try to react with - and damage - other sensitive molecules. The word 'antioxidant' arises from the chemical definitions of 'oxidation' and 'reduction.' A free radical is an 'oxidant,' 'oxidizer' or 'oxidizing agent,' a chemical that wants to take an electron away from another chemical and use that electron to stabilize itself. This damages, or 'oxidizes' the other chemical. An antioxidant is a 'reducer' or a 'reducing agent' that sacrifices one of its electrons to the free radical. When a free radical and an antioxidant react, the free radical is 'reduced' - it has gained an electron; and the antioxidant is 'oxidized' - it has lost an electron. You'd think it would be the other way around...reduction sounds like losing an electron rather than gaining one...but they did it this way just to confuse chemistry students ;>)

Antiseptic

Acting against sepsis. An antiseptic agent is one that has been formulated for use on living tissue such as mucous membranes or skin to prevent or inhibit growth or action of organisms. Antiseptics should not be used to decontaminate inanimate objects.

Antiserum

The blood serum obtained from an animal after has been immunized with a particular antigen. It contains antibodies specific for that antigen as well as antibodies specific for any other antigens with which the animal has previously been immunized.

Antistatic

Reducing static electric charges by retaining enough moisture to provide electrical conduction.

Antistatic Cleaners

Liquid cleaners that enhance surface conductivity of cleanroom tabletops, workstations, and other surfaces.

Antitoxin

An antibody that is capable of neutralizing the specific toxin that stimulated its production in the body. Antitoxins are produced in animals for medical purposes by injection of a toxin or toxoid, with the resulting serum being used to counteract the toxin in other individuals.

Antiviral

An agent or procedure that prevents or inhibits viral infections.

Anti-inflammatory

An agent or procedure that counteracts inflammation.

Anti-interferon

An antibody to an interferon. Used for the purification of interferons.

API (Active Pharmaceutical Ingredient)

Also called Drug Substance. Any substance or mixture of substances intended to be used in the manufacture of a drug (medicinal) product and that when used in the production of a drug becomes an active ingredient of the drug product. Such substances are intended to furnish pharmacological activity or other direct effect in the diagnosis, cure, mitigation, treatment, or prevention of disease or to affect the structure and function of the body.

API Starting Material

A material used in the production of an API which is itself or is incorporated as a significant structural fragment into the structure of the API. A starting material may be an article of commerce, a material purchased from one or more suppliers under contract or commercial agreement, or it may be produced in-house. Starting materials are normally of defined chemical properties and structure.

Apoenzyme

The protein moiety of an enzyme - determines the specifity of the enzyme reaction.

Application Software

Any executable program developed or modified specially for customer applications.

Appropriated login or Impersonation

Someone using the authorization code, usually user ID and password of another person to secure access to network resources for which he or she does not have privileges or authorization. Can be intentional or not. CFR 21 Part 11 mandates technical controls that prevent this.

Aquifer

An underground layer of permeable rock, sand, or gravel that contains water for wells or springs.

Arjuna Bark

Arjuna is the dried bark of *Terminalia arjuna.*

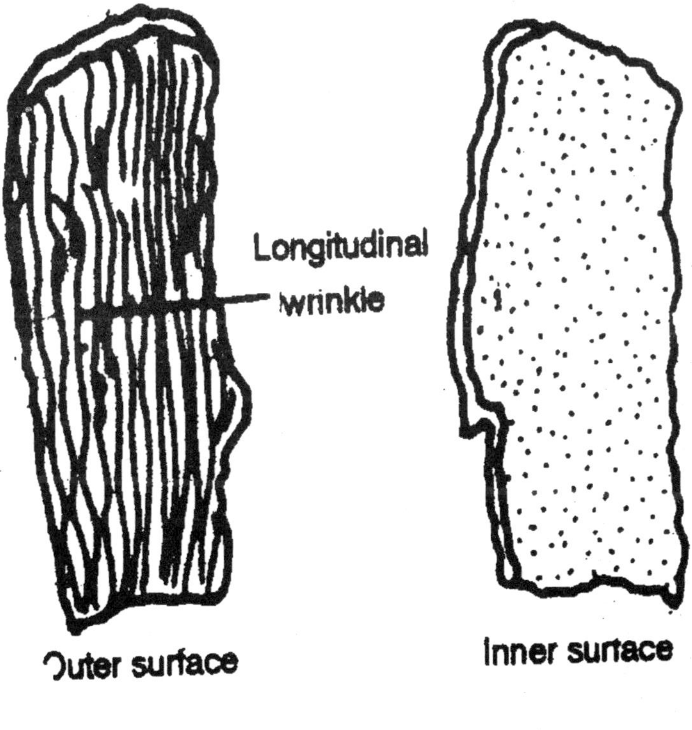

Arjuna Bark

Arithmetic Average Roughness (Ra)

The arithmetic average height of roughness component irregularities from the mean line measured within the sample length (L). This measurement conforms to ANSI/ASME B46.1 "Surface Texture - Surface Roughness, Waviness and Lay". Ra (formerly known as AA or Arithmetic Average in the U.S., and CLA Centerline Average in the U.K.) is usually expressed in microinches (µin), and performed by moving a stylus or profilometer in a straight line along the surface. A consistent and measurable surface finish can be specified for a desired roughness i.e., 9-11 microinch.

Aromatic ring

A structure found in many kinds of phytochemicals, such as phenolic compounds, alkaloids, and terpenes; it consists of six carbon atoms in a flat, hexagonal pattern. It is represented like this:Each angle in the drawing stands for a carbon; the double lines alternating with single lines mean that the atoms are all sharing electrons. In many chemicals, different functional groups (such as -OH or $-CH_3$) are attached to the ring, like this:

(It looks like there are double bonds alternating with single bonds in this ring, but in this special case, there really aren't - all atoms are sharing equally). The aromatic ring got its name from the fact that early chemists discovered it in fragrant substances; but not all phytochemicals containing this structure have an odor.

Asafoetida

Asafoetida, Ferula asafoetida (family Umbelliferae), is a resin gum which comes from the dried sap from the stem and roots of the wild fennel genus Ferula. The resin is greyish-white when fresh, but dries to a dark amber colour. Chunks of asafoetida resin are too hard to be grated easily, and traditionally crushed between stones or with a hammer. Today, the most commonly available form is **compounded asafoetida,** a fine powder containing 30% asafoetida resin, along with rice flour and gum arabic.

It derives its English and scientific name from the Persian word for resin (asa) and Latin foetida, which refers to its strong sulfurous odor. Its pungent odour has resulted in its being called by many unpleasant names; thus the French know it, amongst other names, as Merde du Diable (Devil's faeces); in some dialects of English too it was known as Devil's Dung, and equivalent names can be found in German - Teufels Dreck, Danish - Dyvelsdræk, Dutch - Duivelsdrek, Icelandic - Djöflatað, Norwegian - Dyvelsdrekk, Swedish Dyvelsträck. In Turkish, it is known as ªeytantersi, ªeytan bökösu or ªeytanotu (the Devil's Herb).

In many of the northern Indian languages (Hindi, Urdu, Gujarati, Punjabi, Marathi, Bengali) it is known as hing. In Tamil, it is known as perungaayam. This spice is used as a digestive aid and in pickles. Its odour is so strong that it must be stored in airtight containers; otherwise, it spoils other foodstuffs. It loses its smell in cooking, however, and presents an onion-like taste. In India, it is used especially by the Brahmin caste of the Hindus and by adherents of Jainism, who are not allowed to eat onions. It is mainly grown in Iran, Afghanistan and Kashmir.

It has certain medicinal uses: it aids the digestion, and is helpful in cases of asthma and bronchitis. In the Appalachian region of the United States, it was used as a folk remedy for children's colds: it is mixed into a foul-smelling paste and hung in a bag around the afflicted child's neck.

"As-Built" Cleanroom

ISO 14644-1 defines the "as built" occupancy state as "condition where the installation is complete with all services connected and functioning but with no production equipment, materials, or personnel present".

Ascomycetes

A family of fungi marked by long spore-containing cells. Form sexual spores called ascospores, which are contained within a sac (a capsule structure). Ergot, truffles, some molds of the genera Neurospora and Aspergillus, and yeasts belong to this category.

Ashwagandha

It is the dried roots and stem base of *Withania somnifera.*

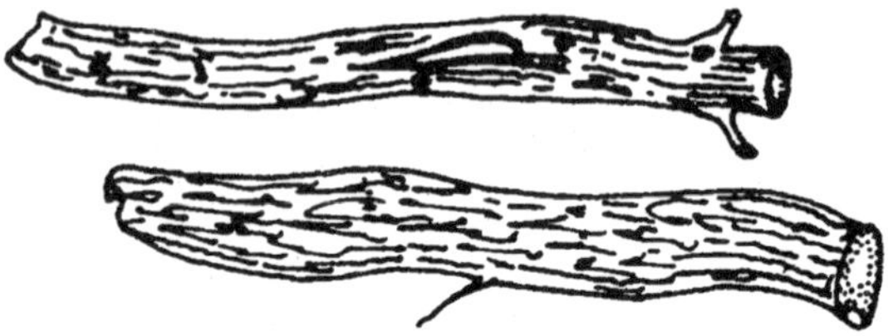

Ashwagandha

Asepsis

A condition in which living pathogenic (causing or capable of causing disease) organisms are absent.

Aseptic

Marked by or relating to asepsis.

Aseptic Processing

Processing conditions designed to achieve a sterile product.

Aseptic Processing Area

Area in which sterile product is formulated, filled into containers, and sealed.

Aseptic Transfer (in Isolators)

The key issue in all contained aseptic environments. Aseptic transfer is essential for change parts, components, and even product to enter and exit an isolator system without sterility challenges. There are an increasing number of ways to make an aseptic transfer. The following is a brief list of some of the key techniques:

1. Alpha Beta Systems Double Door Systems: also called RTPs (Rapid Transfer Ports) and HCT (High Containment Transfer). When mated, the two ports act as one door, protecting the internal and external environments.
2. Alpha Beta Dry Heat Sterilized: similar to Alpha Beta port with the additional safeguard of a heat sterilized seal.
3. UV and Pulsed Light: light sterilization/sanitization. Sterilizing the system by making use of a wide spectrum of

light within the transfer chamber.

4. One Shot Systems: basically, two halves coming together. Similar to an Alpha Beta port but simpler, cheaper, and capable of only a single connection.

5. Heat Welded Bag Systems: passed in or passed out using a continuous polyethylene liner which is heat sealed and cut to maintain the integrity of the internal and external environments.

6. Steam Sterilized: the liquid component or powder path is clean steam sterilized after connection and prior to transfer.

7. Autoclave/Depyrogenation/Dryheat: pass through for batch. Use of conventional autoclave to sterilize a canister provided with an Alpha Beta port and filters to allow the passage of steam and safe aspiration on cooling. Depyrogenation/Dryheat uses dry heat to sterilize and at sufficient temperature depyrogenate components, typically glassware, in a batch oven

8. Depyrogenation Tunnel: standard volume glassware entry. Depyrogenation/Dry heat uses dry heat to sterilize and at sufficient temperature to depyrogenate components, typically glassware, in a tunnel allowing continuous input.

ASME Bioprocessing Equipment (BPE- 1997)

An American National Standard that covers, either directly or by reference, requirements for materials, design, fabrication, examination, inspection, testing, certification (for pressure systems), and pressure relief (for pressure systems) of vessels and piping for bioprocessing systems, including sterility and cleanability (Part SD), dimensions and tolerances (Part DT), surface finish requirements (Part SF), material joining (Part MJ), and equipment seals (Part SG) for the bioprocessing systems in which the pressure vessels and associated piping are involved. This Bioprocessing Equipment (BPE) Standard does not address all aspects of these activities, and those aspects that are not specifically addressed should not be considered prohibited.

Requirements of this Standard apply to:

1. All parts that contact the product, raw materials, and/or product intermediates during manufacturing, process development, or scale-up.

2. All equipment or systems that are critical part of product manufacture, such as Water For Injection (WFI), clean steam, ultrafiltration, intermediate product storage, and centrifuges.

ASME/ANSI B31 Code for Pressure Piping

A number of individually published Sections, each an American National Standard. Rules for each Section reflect the kinds of piping installations considered during its development, as follows:

1. B31.1 Power Piping: piping typically found in electric power generating stations, in industrial and institutional plants, geothermal heating systems, and central and district heating and cooling systems.
2. B31.3 Process Piping: piping typically found in petroleum refineries, chemical, pharmaceutical, textile, paper, semiconductor, and cryogenic plants, and related processing plants and terminals. Certain piping within a facility may be subject to other codes and standards, including but not limited to: (a) ANSI Z223.1 National Fuel Gas Code: piping for fuel gas from the point of delivery to the connection of each fuel utilization device. (b) NFPA Fire Protection Standards: fire protection systems using water, carbon dioxide, halon, foam, dry chemical, and wet chemicals. (c) NFPA 99 Health Care Facilities: medical and laboratory gas systems. (d) Building and plumbing codes, as applicable, for potable hot and cold water, and for sewer and drain systems.
3. B31.4 Pipeline Transportation Systems for Liquid Hydrocarbons and Other Liquids: piping transporting products that are predominately liquids between plants and terminals and within terminals, pumping, regulating, and metering stations.
4. B31.5 Refrigeration Piping: piping for refrigerants and secondary coolants.
5. B31.8 Gas Transportation and Distribution Piping Systems: piping transporting products that are predominately gas between sources and terminals, including compressor, regulating, and metering stations; gas gathering pipelines.
6. B31.9 Building Services Piping: piping typically found in industrial, institutional, commercial, and public buildings, and in multi-unit residences, which does not require the range of sizes, pressures, and temperatures covered in B31.1.
7. B31.11 Slurry Transportation Piping Systems: piping

transporting aqueous slurries between plants and terminals and within terminals, pumping, and regulating stations.

Assay

A technique (test) for measuring a biological response or for determining characteristics such as composition, purity, activity, and weight.

Assimilation

The formation of cellular material utilizing small food molecules and energy.

Astragalus (Astragalus membranaceus)

An immune stimulant thought to inhibit tumor growth and often used to help reduce the side effects of chemotherapy. It supports the production of interferons (proteins our cells produce to fight out viral infections). May be used daily as tonic before colds start.

Atmospheric Tank (Fire Code)

A storage tank designed to operate at pressures from atmospheric through 0.5 pounds per square inch (psig) (3.4 kPa).

Atomic Absorption Spectrophotometry

A highly sensitive instrumental technique for identifying and measuring metals in water.

At Rest

HVAC room condition when unmanned, and without machinery operating. Previously called "static condition".

"At-Rest" Cleanroom

ISO 14644-1 defines "at rest" occupancy state as "condition where the installation is complete with equipment installed and operating in a manner agreed upon by the customer and supplier, but with no personnel present".
European Community (EC) defines "at rest" state as "the condition where the installation is complete with production equipment installed and operating but with no operating

personnel present". The Medicines Inspectorate, however, further clarifies, "It should normally be taken to mean that ventilation systems are operating and other equipment is present in an operational condition but not in use".

Audit Comment

A feature of the audit trail that aids both originator and reviewer in understanding why the originator performed a specific action. CFR 21 Part 11 does not require entering the reason for a record change, but some predicate rules (such as GLPs) do expect an explanation. It is important that the user interface for entering audit comments prevents users from changing the audit trail itself.

Audit Trail

A computer-generated and time-stamped record of who did what, when. CFR 21 Part 11 requires audit trails to be generated independently of operators. An audit trail must capture all activities related to creating, modifying, and destroying records on a system.

Auger Electron Spectroscopy (AES)

An alternative surface analysis that can detect all elements with an atomic number greater than that of helium with the additional ability to analyze sub micron-diameter features. It is not as quantitative as ESCA and cannot determine the chemical state of an element. The primary advantage of Auger is that when combined with etching, a chemical depth profile can be measured rapidly and can image the distribution on the surface of spatial limitation resolution of 100 to 1,000 angstroms (depending on the equipment capability).

Austenite

A face-centered cubic crystal with high solubility for carbon (about 2%); an allotropic form of iron resulting from steel being heated above the transformation temperature.

Autegoneous Weld

A weld made by fusion of the base material without the addition of filler.

Authentication

The process of identifying a person, system, or company sufficiently to allow access to a system or part of a system.

Authentication Mechanisms

Also known as authority checks, or authorized signers are mechanisms distinct from authorization that grants or denies access to a network resource, authentication programs are used by system administrators to establish and verify as conclusively as possible that a person logging in to the network is who he or she claims to be. FDA says that "authority checks" are to "ensure that only authorized individuals can use the system, electronically sign a record, access the operation or computer system, input or output device, alter a record, or perform operations".

Autoclave

An apparatus into which moist heat (steam) under pressure is introduced to sterilize or decontaminate materials placed within (e.g. filter assemblies, glassware, etc.). Steam pressure is maintained for pre-specified times and then allowed to exhaust. There are two types of autoclaves:

1. Gravity displacement autoclave: this type of autoclave operates at 121°C. Steam enters at the top of the loaded inner chamber, displacing the air below through a discharge outlet.
2. Vacuum autoclave: this type of autoclave can operate with a reduced sterilization cycle time. The air is pumped out of the loaded chamber before it is filled with steam.

Auto Immune Disease

A disease in which the body produces an immunogenic response against self-antigens. In some cases, predominantly one organ is affected (e.g. hemolytic anemia and chronic thyroiditis); in others, the disease process is diffused through many tissues (e.g. SLE (Systemic Lupus Erythematosis)).

Automated System

Any facility system or piece of equipment that is controlled with limited or no manual intervention.

Automatic Welding

Welding with equipment that performs the welding operation without adjustment of the controls by a welding operator. The equipment may or may not perform the loading and unloading of the work.

Autoradiography

A technique that uses X-ray film to visualize radioactively labeled molecules or fragments of molecules; used in analyzing length and number of DNA fragments after they are separated by gel electrophoresis.

Autonomic Nervous System

The part of the nervous system that is concerned with involuntary bodily functions.

Autosome

A chromosome not involved in sex determination. The diploid human genome consists of 46 chromosomes, 22 pairs of autosomes, and 1 pair of sex chromosomes.

Autotrophs

One of two categories in which microorganisms are classified on the basis of their carbon source. Autotrophs use carbon dioxide as a carbon source.

BAC (Bacterial Artificial Chromosome)

A vector used to clone DNA fragments (100-kb to 300-kb insert size; average, 150-kb) in E. Coli cells. Based on naturally occurring F-factor plasmid found in the bacterium E. coli.

B

B-Lymphocyte

Lymphoid stem cells from the bone marrow that migrate to and become mature antigen-specific cells in the spleen and lymph nodes. All B cells are antigen specific and respond to only one foreign protein.

Background Contamination

Contamination introduced accidentally in reagents, dilution water, solvents, rinse water, etc., which can be confused with constituents in samples being analyzed.

Background Environment

The environment that surrounds a critical area.

Back-up Copy

A magnetic copy of data, software, user-developed application, or operating parameters associated with an automated system and not considered the original.

Backward Compatibility

A new version of a computer program that can use files and data created with an older version of the same program. A computer is said to be backward compatible if it can run the same software as the previous model. Backward compatibility is important because it eliminates the need to start over when you upgrade to a newer product, but is sometimes sacrificed in favor of a new technology.

Backwash

The countercurrent flow of water through equipment, usually to clean or to recover performance, such as in a resin bed (flow-in at the bottom of the exchanger unit and out at the top) to clean and reclassify the bed after exhaustion. This process of reversing flow may also be applied to filters in order to force contaminants out of plugged pores and passages.

Bacteria

The plural of Bacterium.

Bactericide

An agent that kills vegetative bacteria but not mycobacteria or spores.

Bacteriophage

A virus that exclusively infects bacteria. A protein coat surrounds the genome (DNA or RNA). One of the bacteriophages most extensively studied is the lambda phage, which is also one of the most important viral vectors used in rDNA work. Lambda promoters have been used to express eukaryotic proteins in E.coli.

Bacteriostatic

Inhibiting growth of bacterial organisms without necessarily killing them or their spores.

Bacteriostatic Water

For Injection, U.S.P. Water that serves the same purposes as Sterile Water for Injection, it meets the same standards, with the exception that it may be packaged in either single-dose or multiple-dose containers of not larger than 30-mL size.

Bacterium

Any of a large group of microscopic organisms having round, rod-shaped, spiral, or filamentous unicellular or noncellular bodies that are often aggregated into colonies, are enclosed by a cell wall or membrane (prokaryotes), and lack fully differentiated nuclei. Bacteria range in size from 0.4µm to 2.0µm and may exist as free-living organisms in soil, water, organic matter, or as parasites in the live bodies of plants. Some are disease producing, but most perform necessary functions such as digestion, fermentation, and nitrification. Most of the forms are variously grouped under generic names such as: Alcaligenes, Dialister, Escherichia, Klebsiella, Kurthia, Pasteurella, Salmonella, and Shigella.

Barrier Isolator

A containment device that utilizes barrier technology for the enclosure of a controlled workspace. There are two main types of isolator: 1. Type 1 Isolator: An isolator designed to protect the product from process-generated and external factors that would compromise its quality. 2. Type 2 Isolator: An isolator designed to protect the product from process-generated and external factors that would compromise its quality and to protect the operator from hazards associated with the product.

Barrier Technology

The technology of using separating environments, whether protecting the world from a product or the product from the world. Containment, barrier isolation and isolation all refer to the same technology, which is enclosing an environment. There are, however, some redefining terms that are gaining favor: 1. Containment - protect the world from the product (as in the case of highly potent compounds or a toxic). 2. Isolation - protect the product from the world (as in the case of a sterile product). 3. ISO 14644-7 "Minienvironments and Isolators" will define further levels of devices

Base

An electropositive element or radical that unites with an acid to form a salt. Or, a substance that when dissolved in water, dissociates to produce one or more hydroxyl ions (OH-).

Base Pair (bp)

Two nucleotides that are in different nucleic acid chains and whose bases pair by hydrogen bonding. In DNA, the nucleotide bases are adenine (A) that always pairs with thymine (T) and guanine (G) which pairs with cytosine (C). In RNA molecules, adenine (A) joins the uracil (U). Two strands of DNA are held together in the shape of a double helix by the bonds between these pairs.

Base Sequence

The order of nucleotide bases in a DNA molecule.

Base Sequence

Analysis A method, sometimes automated, for determining the base sequence.

Baseline

In some analytical procedures a sample is dissolved in water or combined with other reagents for analysis. A "blank" or standard consisting of the same reagents may be analyzed without sample present. This provides a comparative reference point, or baseline, so that the test results can be attributed solely to the sample itself.

Baseline® Pharmaceutical Engineering Guides (ISPE)

A series of industry publications developed in partnership with the US Food and Drug Administration (FDA). Each volume in the series is a collaborative effort of industry leaders representing a broad cross-section of manufacturers and other industry experts. The Guides document current industry practice for facilities and systems used for production of pharmaceutical products and medical devices. They are intended to:

- Establish a baseline approach to new and renovated facility design, construction, commissioning, and qualification that is based upon clear understanding of the type of product and its manufacturing process.
- Prioritize facility design features based upon the impact on product and process.
- Avoid unnecessary spending on facility features that do not contribute to consistent production of quality products.

The Guides include five product manufacturing operation based guides (vertical guides), and three support system/ function based guides (horizontal guides):

1. Volume I - Bulk Pharmaceutical Chemicals (1996)
2. Volume II - Oral Solid Dosage Forms (1998)

3. Volume III - Sterile Manufacturing Facilities (1999)
4. Volume VI - Biotech (in progress)
5. Volume -Oral Liquids and Aerosols
6. Volume IV - Water and Steam Systems (in progress)
7. Volume V - Commissioning and Qualification Guide (in progress)
8. Volume VII - Packaging and Warehousing

Basidiomycetes

Reproduce by basidiospores, which are extended from the stalks of specialized cells called the basidia. The class comprises Photobasidiomycetes (smuts and rusts) and the Hymenomycetes (mushrooms and puffballs).

Basis of Design

A design document that describes what the purpose of a given system is and how the system will accomplish its required task. This document is created and approved before the issuance of bid specifications and is often used to develop them. Until the system is developed this is a conceptual document.

Batch

A specific quantity of material produced in a process or series of processes so that is expected to be homogeneous within specified limits. In the case of continuous production a batch may correspond to a defined fraction of the production, characterized by its intended homogeneity. The batch size may be defined either by fixed quantity or the amount produced in a fixed time interval.

Batch Number

A unique combination of numbers and/or letters which specifically identify a batch or lot and from which the production and distribution history can be determined.

Batch Fermentation

The process in which a fixed volume of sterile medium in a vessel is inoculated with a desired organism. The broth is fermented for a defined period to completion, without further additions of media. After discharging the batch, the fermenter is cleaned and rebatched with medium for another cycle. Two other types of fermentation cycles are fed batch and continuous. Batchwise Control The use of validated in-process sampling and testing methods such that results prove the process has done what it purports to do for the specific batch concerned, assuming control parameters have been appropriately maintained.

Bayberry (Myrica ceriferea)

Astringent in diarrhea; reduces secretions; used also in colds and chills; relaxes nervous tension which may be cause colic.

Bay leaf

Bay leaf (plural **bay leaves**) are the aromatic leaves of several species of the Laurel family (Lauraceae). Bay leaves are used in cooking for their distinctive flavor and fragrance, and may be used fresh or dried.

- Mediterranean bay leaf
  The leaf of the bay laurel or "true laurel", *Laurus nobilis*, is a culinary herb often used to flavor soups, stews, and braises and pâtés in Mediterranean Cuisine.
- California bay leaf
  The leaf of the California bay tree (*Umbellularia californica*), also known as 'California laurel', 'Oregon myrtle', and 'pepperwood', is similar to the Mediterranean bay, but has a stronger flavor.
- Indian bay leaf (*Tej pat*)
  The leaf of the *Cinnamomum tejpata* tree, similar in fragrance and taste to cinnamon bark, but milder. In appearance, it is similar to the other bay leaves, but is culinarily quite different.

Bed

Column of carbon, sand, chromatography, or ion exchange resins through which a liquid passes during operation.

Bed Depth

The height of the exchange or capture material in a column after proper backwashing for effective operation.

Bed Expansion

The effect produced during backwashing; resin particles separate and rise in the column. Regulating backwash flow may control bed expansion caused by the increase in space between resin particles.

Belladonna

The drug consist of the leaves and other aerial parts of *Atropa belladonna Linn.* Indian belladonna is obtained from *Atropa acduminata.*

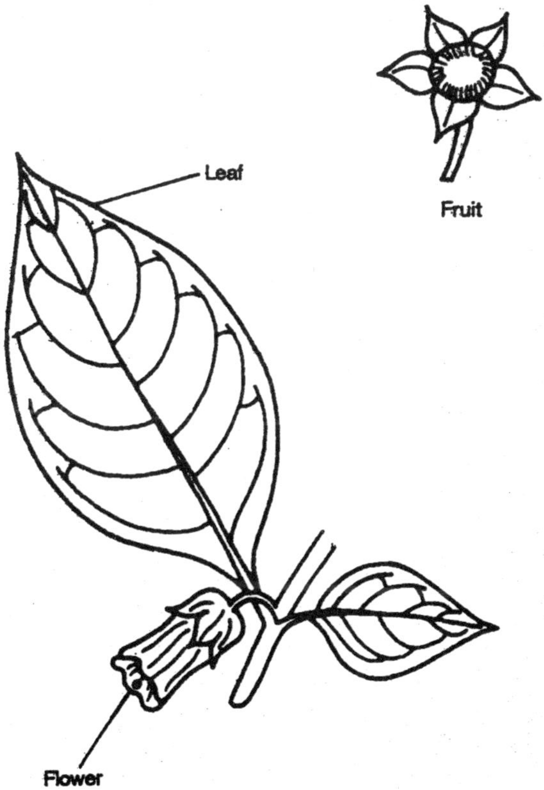

Belladonna

Benzodiazepines

A group of chemically similar psychotropic drugs with potent hypnotic and sedative actions, primarily used as anti-anxiety agents and sedatives.

Berberis

Berberis is a genus of about 450-500 species of deciduous and evergreen shrubs from 1-5 m tall with thorny shoots, native to the temperate and subtropical regions of Europe, Asia, Africa, North America and South America. They are closely related to the genus *Mahonia*, which is included within *Berberis* by some botanists. Many are known by the vernacular name **barberry**. The genus is characterised by dimorphic shoots, with long shoots which form the structure of the plant, and short shoots only 1-2 mm long. The leaves on long shoots are non-photosynthetic, developed into three-spined thorns 3-30 mm long; the bud in the axil of each thorn-leaf then develops a short shoot with several normal, photosynthetic leaves. These leaves are 1-10 cm long, simple, and either entire, or with spiny margins. Only on young seedlings do leaves develop on the long shoots, with the adult foliage style developing after the young plant is 1-2 years old.

The deciduous species (e.g. Berberis thunbergii, B. vulgaris) are noted for good autumn colour, the leaves turning pink or red before falling. In some evergreen species from China (e.g. B. candidula, B. verruculosa), the leaves are brilliant white beneath, making them particularly attractive.

The flowers are produced singly or in racemes of up to 20 on a single flower-head. They are yellow or orange, 3-6 mm long, with six sepals and six petals in alternating whorls of three, the sepals usually coloured like the petals. The fruit is a small berry 5-15 mm long, ripening red or dark blue, often with a pink or violet waxy surface bloom; they may be either long and narrow (like a bar, hence 'barberry') or in other species, spherical. The berries are edible, and rich in vitamin C, though with a very sharp flavour; the thorny shrubs make harvesting them difficult, so they are not widely consumed. They are an important food for many small birds, which disperse the seeds in their droppings.

Several are popular garden shrubs, grown for their ornamental leaves, yellow flowers, and red or blue-black berries. They are also valued for crime prevention; being very dense, viciously spiny shrubs, they make very effective barriers impenetrable to burglars. For this reason they are often planted below potentially vulnerable windows, and used as hedges and other barriers.

Berberis vulgaris, the European Barberry, is the alternate host species of the wheat rust Puccinia graminis, a serious fungal disease of wheat. For this reason, cultivation of this species is prohibited in many areas.

Binary Explosive

An explosive material composed of separate components, each of which is safe for storage and transportation and would not in itself be considered as an explosive.

Binding affinity

A measure of the strength of the attraction and 'sticking power' between a protein (i.e., an estrogen receptor) and its ligand (the molecule which binds to it - i.e., an isoflavone).

Bioaccumulation

The process which results in increasing body burdens of recalcitrant non-water soluble compounds as they move up the food chain.

Bioactivity

A protein's ability to function correctly after it has been delivered to the active site of the body (in vivo).

Bioassay

The determination of the biological activity of a substance (e.g. a drug) by observing its effect on an organism (or organ) compared to a standard preparation.

Bioaugmentation

A strategy involved in bioremediation that increases the activity of an organism to break down or metabolize a pollutant. This involves reseeding a waste site with bacteria as they die.

Bioburden

The level and type of microorganisms which may be present in raw materials, API (Active Pharmaceutical Ingredient) starting materials, intermediates, or APIs which have defined limits and should not affect the quality of the API. Bioburden should not be considered contamination unless the levels have been exceeded or defined objectionable organisms have been detected.

Biochemical Oxygen Demand (BOD)

(also see: BOD (Biochemical Oxygen Demand))

Biochemistry

The study of chemical processes in living things. Despite the dramatic differences in the appearance of living things, the basic chemistry of all organisms is strikingly similar. Even tiny, one-celled creatures carry out essentially the same reactions that each cell of a complex organism, such as man, carries out.

Biocide

An agent that can kill all pathogenic and non-pathogenic living organisms, including spores. More general than bacteriocide, biocide includes insecticides and any compound toxic to any living thing.

Biodegradable

Material that can be broken down by biological action.

Bioequivalency

A scientific basis on which generic and brand name drugs are compared with one another. Drugs are bioequivalent if they enter circulation at the same rate when given in similar doses under similar conditions.

Biodiversity

The number and variety of different organisms in the particular ecological setting.

Biogenerator

A contained system, such as a fermentor, into which biological agents are introduced along with other materials so as to effect their multiplication or their production of other substances by reaction with the other materials. Biogenerators are generally fitted with devices for regulation, control, connection, material addition, and material withdrawal.

Biohazard

An infectious agent(s), or part thereof, presenting a real or potential risk to human, other animals, or plants, directly through infection or indirectly through disruption of the environment.

Bioinformatics

The use of computers in the life sciences, electronic databases of genomes and protein sequences, and computer modeling of biomolecules and biologic systems.

Biologic

A therapeutic agent derived from living things.

Biological Barrier

An impediment (naturally occurring or introduced) to the infectivity and/or survival of a microbiological agent or eukaryotic cell once it has been released into the environment.

Biological Impurities

Impurities resulting from living matter (bacteria, virus, algae, protozoa, microfungi) and their by-products, including pyrogens (endotoxins).

Biological Indicators

Resistant microorganisms placed into or on various materials to confirm that a sterilization process is effective. They may for instance be placed within a filter in order to determine if a proposed autoclave cycle is effective. After autoclave, they are removed and culture tests are performed to see if the microorganisms were killed.

Biological Oxygen Demand (BOD)

(also see: BOD (Biological Oxygen Demand))

Biological Reactivity Tests, In Vivo

This classification is based on responses to a series of in vivo tests for which extracts, materials and routes of administration are specified. Six Plastic Classes are defined:

1. Class I - Uses a specified dosage of an extract of sample in Sodium Chloride Injection applied either intravenously or intracutaneously into a mouse or a rabbit.
2. Class II - Same as Class I but in addition uses an extract of sample in 1 in 20 Solution of Alcohol in Sodium Chloride Injection applied either intravenously or intracutaneously into a mouse or a rabbit.
3. Class III - Same as Class II but in addition uses an extract of sample in Polyethylene Glycol 400, and an extract of sample in Vegetable Oil, both applied either intraperitoneally or intracutaneously into a mouse.
4. Class IV - Same as Class II but in addition uses an extract of sample in Vegetable Oil applied intraperitoneally or intracutaneously into a mouse or a rabbit. Also uses implant strips of sample into a rabbit.
5. Class V - Same as Class II but in addition uses an extract of sample in Polyethylene Glycol 400, and an extract of sample in Vegetable Oil applied intraperitoneally or intracutaneously into a mouse or a rabbit.
6. Class VI - Same as Class V but in addition uses implant strips of sample into a rabbit.

These tests are designed to determine the biological response of animals to elastomerics, plastics and other polymeric material with direct or indirect patient contact, or by the injection of specific extracts prepared from the material under test. Three tests are described:

1. Systemic Injection Test - Designed to determine the systemic biological responses of animals to plastics and other polymers by the single-dose injection of specific extracts prepared from a sample.
2. Intracutaneous Test - Designed to determine the local biological responses of animals to plastics and other polymers by the single-dose injection of specific extracts prepared from a sample.

3. Implantation Test - Designed to evaluate the reaction of living tissue to the plastic and other polymers by the implantation of the sample (specimen under test) itself into animal tissue. With the exception of the Implantation Test, the procedures are based on the use of extracts that, depending on the heat resistance of the material, are prepared at one of the three standard temperatures: 50°, 70°, and 121°. Therefore, the class designation of a plastic must be accompanied by an indication of the temperature of extraction e.g., IV - 121°, which represents a class IV plastic extracted at 121°).

Biological Safety Cabinets (BSCs)

Bench-top or freestanding cabinets with unidirectional airflow used for handling materials that present a health hazard. The National Institutes of Health (NIH) Guidelines classify them as:

1. Class I - A negative pressure, ventilated cabinet for personnel protection having an inward flow of air away from the operator. The exhaust air is filtered through a HEPA filter (located at rear or top) either into the laboratory or to the outside. This cabinet is designed for general microbiological research with low and moderate risk agents (BL-2 and BL-3 agents), and is used in three operational modes:

a) With a full width open front. The face velocity of the inward flow of air through the full width open front is at least 75' feet per minute.

b) With an installed front closure panel (having four 6-inch diameter openings) without gloves. The face velocity of the inward flow of air through the openings will increase to approximately 150' feet per minute.

c) With an installed front closure panel equipped with arm-length rubber gloves, and inlet air pressure relief for further protection. In this configuration, it is necessary to install a make-up air inlet fitted with a HEPA filter in the cabinet.

2. Class II - A ventilated cabinet for personnel and product protection having an open front with inward airflow for personnel protection (75' to 100' feet per minute), and HEPA filtered downward unidirectional airflow for product protection. The exhaust air is filtered through a HEPA filter for environmental protection. For selection and procurement

of Class II cabinets refer to standards developed by the National Sanitation Foundation, Ann Arbor, Michigan. Cabinets are further classified as:

a) Type A - Suitable for microbiological research in the absence of volatile or toxic chemicals and radionuclides (BL-2 and BL-3), with 70% recirculated air through HEPA. They are exhausted through HEPA into the laboratory or to the outdoors via a "thimble" connection to the building exhaust system.

b) Type B - Hard ducted to the building exhaust system, contains negative pressure plena, and face velocity of 100' feet per minute. Type B cabinets are further sub-typed into types: B1 (30% recirculated air through HEPA; exhaust via HEPA and hard ducted. BL2 and BL-3), B2 (No recirculation; total exhaust via HEPA and hard ducted. BL-2 and BL-3), and B3 (same as IIA, but plena under negative pressure to room and exhaust air is ducted. BL-2 and BL-3).

Classes I and II should be located away from traffic patterns and doors, airflow from fans, room air supply louvers, and other air moving devices.

3. Class III - Closed-front ventilated cabinet of gas tight construction that provides the highest level of personnel protection from infectious aerosols, as well as protection of research materials from microbiological contaminants. The interior of the cabinet is protected from contaminants exterior to the cabinet. The cabinet is fitted with arm-length rubber gloves and is operated under negative pressure of at least 0.5 inches water gauge. All supply air is filtered through HEPA filters. Exhaust air is filtered through two HEPA filters in series or one HEPA filter and incinerator before being discharged to the outside environment. Class III cabinets are most suitable for work with hazardous agents that require Biosafety Level 3 or 4 containment. Cabinets must be connected to a double-door autoclave and/or chemical dunk tank used to sterilize or disinfect all materials exiting the cabinet, and to allow supplies to enter the cabinet.

Biologics

"Any virus, therapeutic serum, toxin, antitoxin, vaccine, blood, blood component or derivative, allergenic product, or analogous product... applicable to the prevention, treatment, or cure of diseases or injuries of man..."

Biomass

Organic matter grown by the photosynthetic conversion of solar energy.

Biomass

The entire assemblage of living organisms (both plant and animal), of a particular region, considered collectively.

Biometabolism

Physical and chemical processes that occur within a cell or an organism, for example, the conversion of nutrients into energy.

Biometrics

A method of verifying an individual's identity based on measurement of his/her physical feature(s) or repeatable action(s) where those features and/or actions are both measurable and unique to that individual. The main types of biometrics are: face recognition, finger scanning, hand geometry, finger geometry, iris recognition, palm, retina, signature, and voice recognition.

Bionics

An interscience discipline for constructing artificial systems, which resemble or have the characteristics of living systems.

Biopharmaceuticals

Ethical pharmaceutical drugs derived through bioprocessing.

Bioprocessing

The creation of a product utilizing a living organism.

Bioprocess Engineering

Process that uses complete living cells or their components (e.g., enzymes, chloroplast) to effect desired physical or chemical changes.

Biopsy

The gross and microscopic examination of tissues or cells removed from a living patient, for the purpose of diagnosis or prognosis of disease, or for the confirmation of normal conditions.

Biopure Water

Water that is sterile, pyrogen free and has a total solids content of less than 1 ppm.

Biosphere

All the living matter on or in the earth, the oceans and seas, and the atmosphere.

Bioreactor

A closed system used for bioprocessing (flask, roller bottle, tank, vessel, or other container), which supports the growth of cells, mammalian or bacterial, in a culture medium. A bacterial reaction usually is said to take place in a fermenter, and cell culture in a bioreactor.

Biosafety Level

The National Institutes of Health (NIH) specifies physical containment levels and defines Biosafety Levels in their "Guidelines for Research Involving Recombinant DNA Molecules" - Appendix G - May 1999. There are four biosafety levels for operations performed with infectious agents:

1. BL1: Practices, safety equipment, and facilities appropriate for work performed with defined and characterized strains of viable microorganisms not known to cause disease in healthy adult humans. The Basic Laboratory. This laboratory provides general space in which work is done with viable agents that are not associated with disease in healthy adults. Conventional laboratory designs are adequate. Areas known to be source of general contamination, such as animal rooms and waste staging areas, should not be adjacent to patient care activities. Public areas and general offices to which non-laboratory staff requires frequent access should be separated from spaces, that primarily support laboratory functions.

2. BL2: Practices, safety equipment, and facilities appropriate for work performed with a broad spectrum of moderate risk agents present and associated with human disease of varying severity. The Basic Laboratory. This laboratory provides

general space in which work is done with viable agents that are not associated with disease in healthy adults. Conventional laboratory designs are adequate. Areas known to be sources of general contamination, such as animal rooms and waste staging areas, should not be adjacent to patient care activities. Public areas and general offices to which non-laboratory staff requires frequent access should be separated from spaces, which primarily support laboratory functions.

3. BL3: Practices, safety equipment, and facilities appropriate for work performed with indigenous or exotic agents where the potential for infection by aerosols is real and the disease may have serious or lethal consequences. Just walking through the area and breathing the air could infect one. The Containment Laboratory. This laboratory has special engineering features that make it possible for laboratory workers to handle hazardous materials without endangering themselves, the community, or the environment. The unique features that distinguish this laboratory from the basic laboratory are the provisions for access control and a specialized ventilation system. The containment laboratory may be an entire building, a single module, or complex of modules within a building. In all cases, a controlled access zone from areas open to the public separates the laboratory.

4. BL4: Practices, safety equipment, and facilities appropriate for work performed with dangerous and exotic agents that pose a high individual risk of life-threatening disease. Exposure to the skin could cause infection. The Maximum Containment Laboratory. This laboratory has special engineering and containment features that allow activities involving infectious agents that are extremely hazardous to the laboratory worker or that may cause serious epidemic disease to be conducted safely. Although the maximum containment laboratory is generally a separate building, it can be constructed as an isolated area within the building. The laboratory's distinguishing characteristic is that it has secondary barriers to prevent hazardous materials from escaping into the environment. Such barriers include sealed openings into the laboratory, airlocks or liquid disinfectant barriers, a clothing-change and shower room contiguous to the laboratory, a double door autoclave, a biowaste treatment system, and a treatment system to decontaminate exhaust air.

Biosynthesis

The production, by biological synthesis or degradation, of compounds by a living organism (e.g. amino acid synthesis, nucleotide synthesis).

Biosynthesized

A molecule is biosynthesized if it is made by living systems (plants, animals, etc); as opposed to laboratory synthesis.

Biotechnology

An industry that creates, develops, and markets a variety of techniques that use living organisms, or substances from those organisms, to make or modify a product by microbial and biochemical processes. A common misconception is that biotechnology refers only to recombinant DNA or gene splicing work. Recombinant DNA is only one of the many techniques used to derive products for organisms, plants, and parts of both for the biotechnology industry. A list of areas covered by the term biotechnology would more properly include: plant tissue culture, cell fusion techniques (especially for the production of monoclonal antibodies), enzyme systems, plant breeding, meristem culture, fermentation, and others.

Biotechnology

A process of applying genetic engineering (recombinant DNA), hybrid (monoclonal antibody), hybridization (gene probes), bioelectric, etc. to commercial applications in pharmaceutical, chemical, medical diagnostic device, food, animal and plant industries.

Biotechnology

Products Large molecules that are not manufactured by means of chemical synthesis but rather produced by means of fermentation and/or recovery, sourced from genetically engineered products.

Biowaste Inactivation

The inactivation or "killing" of biological organisms using heat or chemicals. This step is done at the end of the processing to ensure that there are no living organisms remaining in the effluent that is sent to the sanitary sewer system. Heat is usually applied at 130°C (266°F) for mammalian cells. Chemicals used include caustic or acid.

BLA (Biologics License Application)
The required application for marketing a biologic product in the United States. Most biopharmaceuticals are biologics.

Black cardamom

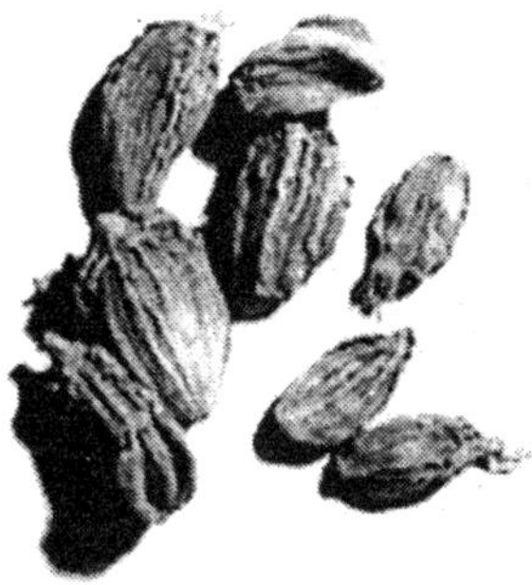

Black cardamom (Amomum subulatum), also known as Brown cardamom or Nepal cardamom, like cardamom is in the Zingiberaceae. It is used in the same way as the green Indian cardamom, but has a drastically different flavor so is not a substitute in the same recipes.

Black Cohosh (Cimacifuga racemosa)
An emmenagogue; assists in balancing female hormones and regulating menstrual periods12; used as an anti-inflammatory in arthritis13; helps lower high blood pressure14; sometimes induces labor and regulates contractions.

Black cumin
The English common name Black Cumin is usually used for Nigella sativa L. but also, less commonly for Bunium persicum [Boiss.] B. Fedtsch of the family Apiaceae.
Nigella sativa (Hebrew, kezah; Arabic, habbah elbaraka, literally seeds of blessing, Persian ÓíÇåÏÇäå siyah daneh, Hindi kalonji) is a spice that grows wild in the Mediterranean

region and in Western Asia. In English it is also called fennel flower, black caraway, nutmeg flower or Roman coriander. It is also sometimes just referred to as Nigella or black seeds. It belongs to the Ranunculaceae family and is unrelated to common cumin (Cuminum cyminum).

Nigella is an annual herbaceous plant that grows to about a foot high. It has a thin stem, narrow (but not filiform) leaflets, and blue flowers. The seeds (the part used) are contained in an inflated capsule formed from the united follicles.

Nigella has a pungent bitter taste and a faint smell of strawberries. It is used primarily in candies and liquors. In herbal medicine, Nigella has hypertensive, carminative, and anthelminthic properties.

Black Haw (Viburnum prunifolium)

Believed to tone the female reproductive system; helps prevent threatened miscarriage15; contains uterine muscle relaxants16.

Black pepper

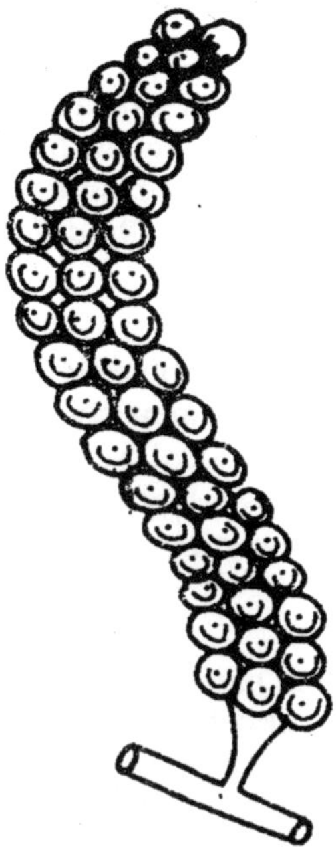

Black pepper

Black pepper consists of the dried unripe fruits of *Piper nigrum*.

Black Walnut (Juglans nigra)

Used in gargles for sore throat; a vermifuge17; a blood purifier; lowers blood pressure.

Blank

A preliminary analysis omitting only the sample to provide an unbiased reference point or baseline for comparison. It is important to minimize extraneous contamination that could be confused with constituents in the sample itself.

Blind Weld

A "blind weld" is defined as a pipe or tube joint welded automatically in which there is no physical way to inspect the weld either visually or with a borescope.

Blinding Clinical trial technique in which, to eliminate bias in a research study, subjects and/or clinical investigators remain unaware of which investigational product is provided.

Blood-Borne Pathogens

Infectious microorganisms that are carried in the blood of infected humans or animals and that can be transmitted through contact with infected blood, body fluids, tissues, or organs. Blood-borne pathogens are implicated in diseases such as malaria, syphilis, brucellosis, tuberculosis, hepatitis B, and AIDS (Acquired Immunodeficiency Syndrome). Workplace transmission of a blood-borne pathogen can occur via accidental inoculation with a contaminated "sharp" exposure through open cuts, skin abrasions, and mucous membranes of eyes and mouth indirect transmission (e.g., touching mouth, eyes, nose or open cuts with contaminated hands).

Blood-brain barrier

A barrier membrane between circulating blood and the brain, preventing some substances from reaching brain tissue and cerebrospinal fluid.

Blood Corpuscle

A cell that circulates in the blood.

Blood Plasma

Blood from which all blood corpuscles, with the exception of platelet cells, have been removed (e.g. by centrifugation) resulting in a clear, straw-colored fluid, which clots as easily as whole blood.

Blood Plateiets

Small, disc-shaped, metabolically active cells circulating in the blood. They are essential in the blood clotting process since they aggregate to form a plug on the injured surface of the blood vessel.

Blood Serum

The liquid expressed from clotted blood or clotted blood plasma.

Blowdown

The bleeding-off of fixed quantities of accumulated feed water to reduce concentrated impurities. If these impurities are permitted to accumulate, they may pass through the distillation process and contaminate the distillate or foul the distillation system.

Blowdown

The withdrawal of water from an evaporating water system to maintain a solids balance within specified limits of concentration of those solids.

Blow (Form) Fill, Seal

Refers to machines that combine formation of a plastic container by blow molding, aseptic filling of a liquid product and sealing of the final package. In the U.S., a major company is ALP, or Automatic Liquid Packaging (Weiler Engineering) and in Europe, Rommilog.

Blue Cohosh (Caulophyllum thalactroides)

Antispasmodic (an agent that relaxes nervous tension that may cause colic); emmenagogue; used to diminish menstrual cramps; used for uterine inflammation and uterine toning;

assists in "false labor" (contractions that don't lead to birth) and helps prevent miscarriage; assists in labor.

BME (Basic Medium Eagles)

One of the most common tissue culture media composed of isotonic salts, carbohydrates and vitamins. When combined with animal serum. BME is a good medium for cell proliferation.

BOD (Biochemical Oxygen Demand)

The amount of oxygen required to oxidize the dissolved organic matter in a water sample by aerobic (bacterial) decay. A measure of the oxygen depletion that would result from discharging organic impurities into a waterway.

BOD (Biological Oxygen Demand)

The oxygen used in meeting the metabolic needs of aerobic organisms in water containing organic compounds.

Bond (covalent bond)

When atoms in the molecules we discuss here are bonded, they are sharing one or more pairs of electrons, and maintain a particular relationship in space to one another. When only one pair is shared, it's a single bond. When two pairs are shared, you have a double bond. See also Hydrogen bond.

Boneset (Eupatorium perfolatum)

Diaphoretic; helps reduce fevers; bitter action for liver, gall bladder, and bowel.

Borage (Borago officinalis)

Lactagoge; diaphoretic; anti-inflammatory; lowers fevers during convalescence.

BPC (Bulk Pharmaceutical Chemical)

A pharmaceutical product derived by chemical synthesis, in bulk form, for later dispensing, formulation or compounding, and filling in a pharmaceutical finishing facility.

Breakthrough Passage of a substance through a bed, filter, or process designed to eliminate it. For ion exchange processes, the first signs are leakage of ions (in mixed beds, usually Silica) and the resultant increase in conductivity. For organic removal beds, usually small, volatile compounds (Trihalomethanes (THMs) are common in activated carbon).

Braze Welding

A welding process using nonferrous filler metal that has a melting point below that of the base metals, but above 427°C (800°F). The filler metal is not distributed in the joint by capillary attraction. This type of welding has been also called Bronze welding, a misnomer.

Brazing

A metal joining process wherein coalescence is produced by use of a nonferrous filler metal having a melting point above 427°C (800°F), but lower than that of the base metals being joined. The filler metal is distributed between the closely fitted surfaces of the joint by capillary action.

Breath Control Shields

Typically made of acrylic or plastic materials, shields protect product, equipment, or the work from particulate contamination expelled by people.

Broad Spectrum

Over a wide range. A broad-spectrum disinfectant is effective against a wide range of microorganisms including bacterial spores, mycobacteria, non-lipid and lipid viruses, fungi, and vegetative bacteria.

Broad spectrum extract

An herbal extract designed to contain a wide range of the compounds found in the original plant, as opposed to a narrow spectrum extract, which focuses on achieving high levels of only one or a few compounds.

Broth

The liquid culture medium in which fermentation or cell culture takes place.

Breakthrough

The first appearance in the effluent of an ion-exchange unit of unadsorbed components similar to those that deplete the activity of the resin bed. Breakthrough indicates that the resin is exhausted and needs to be regenerated.

BSE (Bovine Serum Albumin)

A blood protein that makes up approximately 55-65% of the proteins in the bovine serum. Used as a size marker on gels and as carrier protein.

BSE (Bovine Spongiform Encephalopathy)

Sometimes called "Mad Cow Disease". A disease of cattle presumably caused by a virus or other unidentified entity that affects the brain and causes the cow to behave erratically. Prevalent in parts of Europe but not in the United States. BSE is a contaminant that is undesirable in bovine sera. It is not known whether the causative agent can be filtered out since the causative agent itself is not known. In humans, it is believed to cause Creutzfeld-Jacob, a disease affecting the nervous system.

Btu (British thermal unit)

The unit used to measure the amount of heat in a substance. One Btu is the heat required to produce a temperature rise of 1°F. in one lb. of water.

Bubble Point Test

A filter leakage test in which the filter is wetted and air pressure is applied and slowly increased until water is expelled from the largest pores and bubbles appear from a submerged tube in a downstream collection vessel. Vigorous bubbling, as opposed to a diffusional airflow or occasional bubbles, is indicative of reaching the bubble point. This visual test can be fairly accurate for low area filters, such as discs. When used to evaluate high area filters, it is subject to limitations in observation, test time, collection conditions, and pressurization rates. The bubble point test is not recommended for integrity testing of filter cartridges.

Buchu (Barosma betulina)

Diuretic; reduces inflamed mucous membranes that cause a mucous discharge; helps heal cystitis (infection of the urinary bladder and tract) and prostatis (infection of the prostrate gland); relieves irritation of the bladder, kidneys, urethra18.

Buffer

A substance capable of neutralizing both acids and bases in solution, thereby maintaining the original acidity or causticity of the solution.

Buffer Prep

Area Section of most biotech facilities devoted to the preparation of controlled bioburden buffer solutions for use in the chromatographic separation area of those facilities.

Building Occupancy Classification (California Building Code)

Every building, whether existing or to be erected, is classified by the building official according to its use or the character of its occupancy. The occupancy groups are as follows:

1. Group A - Assembly (Section 303.1.1)
2. Group B - Business (Section 304.1)
3. Group C - Organized Camp (Section 431A)
4. Group E - Educational (Section 305.1)
5. Group F - Factory and Industrial (Section 306.1)
6. Group H - Hazardous (Section 307.1) (also see: Hazardous Occupancy - Group H)
7. Group I - Institutional (Section 308.1)
8. Group M - Mercantile (Section 309.1)
9. Group R - Residential (Section 310.1)
10. Group S - Storage (Section 311.1)
11. Group U - Utility (Section 312.1)

Bulk Handling

The transferring of flammable or combustible liquids from tanks or drums into smaller containers for distribution.

Bulk Oxygen System

An assembly of equipment, such as storage containers, pressure regulators, safety devices, vaporizers, manifolds, and interconnecting piping that has a storage capacity of more than 12,000 cubic feet (340 m^3) of oxygen at normal temperature and pressure, connected in service or ready for service, or more than 25,000 cubic feet (708 m^3) of oxygen, including unconnected reserve on hand at the site.

Bulk Pharmaceutical Chemical (BPC)
(also see: BPC (Bulk Pharmaceutical Chemical))

Burdock Root (Arctium lappa)
Stimulates appetite and digestion; reduces arthritic pain; blood purifier19; treats scrofula, and other cankerous skin conditions20; Burdock root also combined with dandelion and yellow dock can cure a the swelling of a sore growing on top of a lip21.

Butternut Bark (Juglans cinera)
eliminates intestinal worms; a mild laxative22; increases secretion of bile and activity of glands in the walls of the intestinal tract23.

BVD (Bovine Viral Diarrhea)
Viral contaminant found in bovine sera. Able to be filtered out using 0.1 µm nylon filters.
Bovine Of, relating to, or from a cow: such as Bovine Blood: blood from a cow.

Byte
An abbreviation for binary term. A storage unit capable of holding eight bits or the space required for a single letter or number, a single character.

C

Caffeic acid

Also known as 3,4-dihydroxycinnamic acid, caffeic acid is a cinnamic acid derivative that is found in plants.

Calcium

A metallic dyad element of a lustrous yellow color, symbol Ca, atomic number 20, atomic weight 40.09, melting point 810°, often found in water usually as dissolved calcium carbonate, chalk ($CaCO_3$). Soluble in water, it causes hardness and subsequent scaling.

Calcium Carbonate Equivalent

The value obtained when salts are calculated in terms of equivalent quantities of calcium carbonate. This is a convenient method of reducing all salts to a common basis for comparison.

$$\text{ppm } CaCO_3 = \text{ppm ion X } \frac{\text{Equivalent weight of } CaCO_3}{\text{Equivalent weight of ion}}$$

Where ion = magnesium, calcium, or other elements that contribute to hardness.

Calibration

A comparison of a measurement standard or instrument of unknown accuracy to detect, correlate, report, or eliminate by adjustment of any variation in the accuracy of the unknown standard or instrument.

Calibration (ICH API defintion)

The demonstration that a particular instrument or device produces results within specified limits by comparison with those produced by a reference or traceable standard over an appropriate range of measurements.

Calorie

Any of several approximately equal units of heat, each measured as the quantity of heat required to raise the temperature of one (1) gram of water by °C from a standard initial temperature, specially from 3.98°C, 14.5°C, or 19.5°C, at a constant pressure of one (1) atmosphere. Also called "gram calorie", "small calorie".

The unit of heat equal to 1/100 the quantity of heat required to raise the temperature of one (1) gram of water from 0°C to 100°C at one (10 atmosphere pressure. Also called "mean calorie".

The unit required to raise the temperature of one (1) Kilogram of water by 1°C at one (1) atmosphere pressure. Also called "kilogram calorie", "large calorie".

Calorimetry

Analytical method that measures heat loss or gain resulting from physical or chemical changes in a sample. Differential scanning calorimetry compares the results of heating a sample to those for heating a reference material. For example, a method to measure the temperature at which the sample crystallizes, changes phases, or decomposes.

Cancer

The name given to a group of diseases that are characterized by uncontrolled cellular growth.

Candlenut

The ***candlenut, candleberry, Indian walnut, varnish tree*** or ***kuku'i nut tree,*** **Aleurites moluccana** *(Family Euphorbiaceae) is native to Malesia.*

Its native range is impossible to establish precisely because of early spread by man, and the tree is now widely distributed in the new and old world tropics. The tree grows to a height of up to 20 m (60 ft), and is ornamental, with widespreading or pendulous branches bearing pale green leaves. The nut is roundish, and furrowed, about 2 (1-4) cm in diameter, and the seed inside has a very hard seed coat and has a high oil content.

The candlenut has many uses:

- It is often used in Malaysian cuisine.
- Several parts of the plant have been used in traditional medicine in most of the areas where it is native. The oil is an irritant and purgative and sometimes used like castor oil; it has also been used as a hair stimulant. The seed kernels have a laxative effect. In Japan its bark has been used on tumors. In Sumatra, pounded seeds, burned with charcoal, are applied around the navel for costiveness. In Malaya, the pulped kernels or boiled leaves are used in poultices for headache, fevers, ulcers, swollen joints, and gonorrhea. In Java, the bark is used for bloody diarrhea or dysentery.
- In ancient Hawai'i, nuts were burned to provide light. This led to their use as a measure of time. The nuts were strung in a row on a palm leaf midrib and one end lit. One could then instruct someone to return home before the second nut burned out.

In Hawai'i—kuku'i is the Hawaiian name—the tree has spiritual significance of hope and renewal, and was involved in many legends. One such was about a woman who, despite her best efforts to please her husband, was routinely beaten. Finally, the husband beat her to death and buried her under a kuku'i tree. Being a kind and just woman, she was given new life, and the husband was eventually killed.

Modern cultivation is mostly for the oil. In plantations, each tree will produce 30–80 kg of nuts, and the nuts yield 15 to 20% of their weight in oil. Most of the oil is used locally rather than figuring in international trade.

Cannabis

Cannabis consists of dried flowering tops of pistillate plants of *Cannabis sativa* Linn.

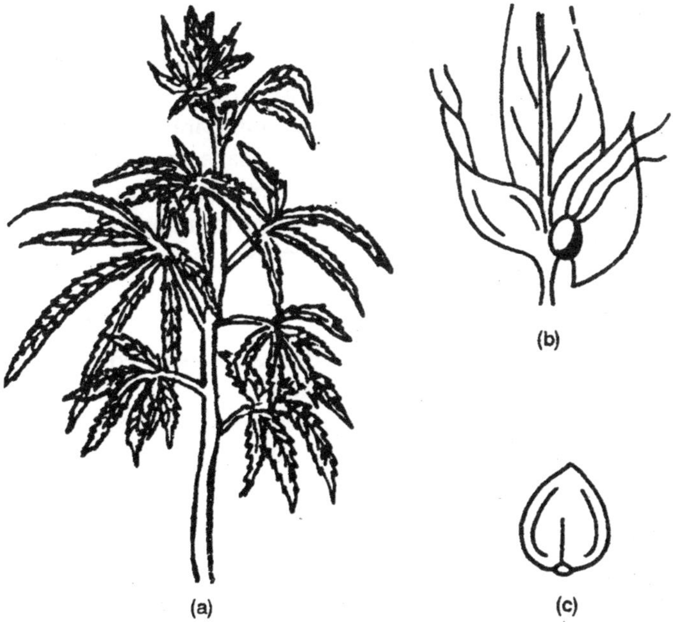

(a) Cannabis herb (b) Bract and bracteole opened to show flower (c) Fruit of cannabis

Caper

A Caper *(Capparis spinosa)* is a shrub from the Mediterranean region. It is best known for its edible buds and fruit which are usually consumed pickled.

Capsid

The external protein shell or coat of a virus particle.

Caraway

Caraway** or **Persian cumin **(Carum carvi)** is a plant that belong to the Apiaceae, or parsley, family. Its seeds is used as a spice, in breads, liquors, casseroles, and other foods, especially in

Central European and Scandinavian cuisine, for instance Sauerkraut. It is also used to add flavour to cheeses. Several liqueurs are made with caraway.

Caraway seeds are crescent-shaped and around 2 millimeters long, with five pale ridges. The seed, usually used whole, has a pungent, anise-like flavor. The aroma comes from essential oils, mostly carvone and limonene. Caraway seed oil is also used as a fragrance component in soaps, creams and perfumes. The plant looks similar to a carrot plant, with finely divided leaves. It has white or pink flowers in umbels. The roots may be cooked like parsnips or carrots.

Carbohydrates

A large class of carbon-hydrogen-oxygen compounds that includes the sugars and their polymers (mainly starch, glycogen and cellulose). Most carbohydrates are produced by photosynthesis in plants. They are the major food compounds for both plants and animals. One group of carbohydrates, cellulose, is the primary structural material of plants.

Carbohydrates and Related Compounds

Plant energy storage components are referred to as carbohydrates. The group which the term carbohydrates represents includes mono- (sucrose, lactose, etc.), and poly- (starch, inulin) saccharides, some acids which are produced after cellular carbohydrate respiration, alcohols such as sorbitol and cellulose; and gums and mucilages. For the purposes of therapeutics, usually the polysaccharide and gum/mucilage subgroups are most important.

Polysaccharides are known to exert a beneficial action on the body's immune system, increasing its strength. They are produced through the linkage of simple or single sugars linked by ethers in various and complex ways, and are divided into two categories, water soluble or water non-soluble. Plant starch, gums, mucilage, cellulose (and sub-group hemicellulose) are all polysaccharides.

Cellulose, i.e., cotton, powdered cellulose, microcrystalline cellulose, and purified rayon, is another polysaccharide, whose derivatives, have been developed as bulking agents for the alleviation of constipation, as opthalmic solutions, topical emollients and protectants, and as agents meant to reduce the appetite.

It has been difficult for phytochemists to distinguish between gums and mucilage categorically. Presently, it is generally agreed that while gums are water solvent, mucilage will become a slimy mass; and, that gums are pathologically formed while mucilages are physiological in origin.

Mucilage, therapeutically, can reduce bowel irritation, gut irritation, peristalsis, toxin absorption, cough, bronchial and urinary spasm. Mucilage can also increase expectoration (Cabrera, 35). As a gelating agent, the polysaccharide hydrocolloidal carrageenan often finds its way in ice cream; it is also used as a laxative ingredient. Perhaps the most common bulking agent derived from a polysaccharide comes from Plantago major, whose seed, the psyllium, can bulk itself up with the addition of water sufficiently to initiate peristalsis and evacuate the bowels.

Carbonyl group

An oxygen atom double-bonded to a carbon atom.

Carbon Filter

A vessel loaded with activated carbon and used to remove organics, chlorine, tastes, and odors from liquids, operating on the principle of adsorption.

Carbon Thickness

A measurement of surface organic material. Carbon thickness values typically range from 5 to 20 angstroms (Å). Significantly contaminated surfaces can show surface carbon thickness of 20 angstroms (Å) or more.

Carbonate Hardness

That hardness in water caused by bicarbonates and carbonates of calcium and magnesium. If alkalinity exceeds total hardness, all hardness is carbonate hardness; if hardness exceeds alkalinity, the carbonate hardness equals the alkalinity.

Carcinogen

A substance that causes the development of cancerous growths in living tissue. A chemical is considered to be a carcinogen if it has been evaluated by the International Agency for Cancer Research (IARC) and found to be a carcinogen or potential carcinogen, or if it is listed in the Annual Report on Carcinogens published by the National Toxicology Program, or if it is regulated by OSHA as a carcinogen.

Carcinogenic

Cancer-causing. Many agents that are carcinogenic are mutagens.

Cardamom

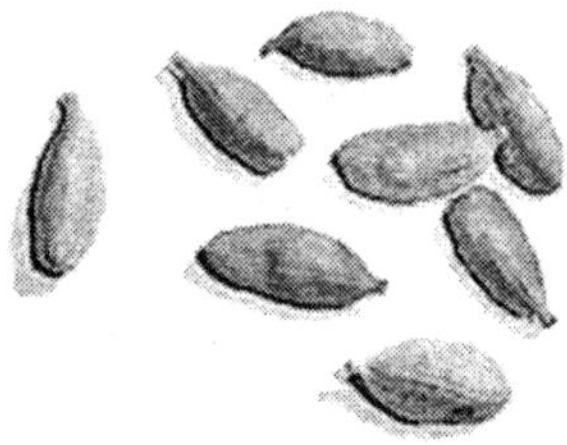

Cardamom fruit as used as spice.

Cardamom *(Elettaria cardamomum)* is a pungent aromatic spice belonging to the family Zingiberaceae. It is a perennial plant that can grow to be between six and 12 feet tall. Cardamom can also be spelt Cardamon, and in India it is popularly known as **elaichi**.

The green seed pods of the plant are dried and the seeds inside the pod are used in Indian and Asian cuisine either whole or in a ground form. Ground Cardamom is a primary ingredient of curry powder. In the Middle East, Cardamom is used for coffee; in other countries such as Iran, it is used to flavor tea. Cardamom is also an ingredient of herbal teas from India, called "Yogi tea." The Indian state of Sikkim has the highest area under cultivation and production of the spice in India.

Cardamom was first used around *700 CE* and was imported to Europe for the first time in around 1200. Originally from the tropical rainforest of India, Sri Lanka, Malaysia and Sumatra, it is now also grown in Nepal, Thailand, and Central America. Cardamom has a strong, pungent taste, with a fragrance reminiscent of eucalyptus oil, while being more complex and subtle. It is often used in Danish pastry and breads.

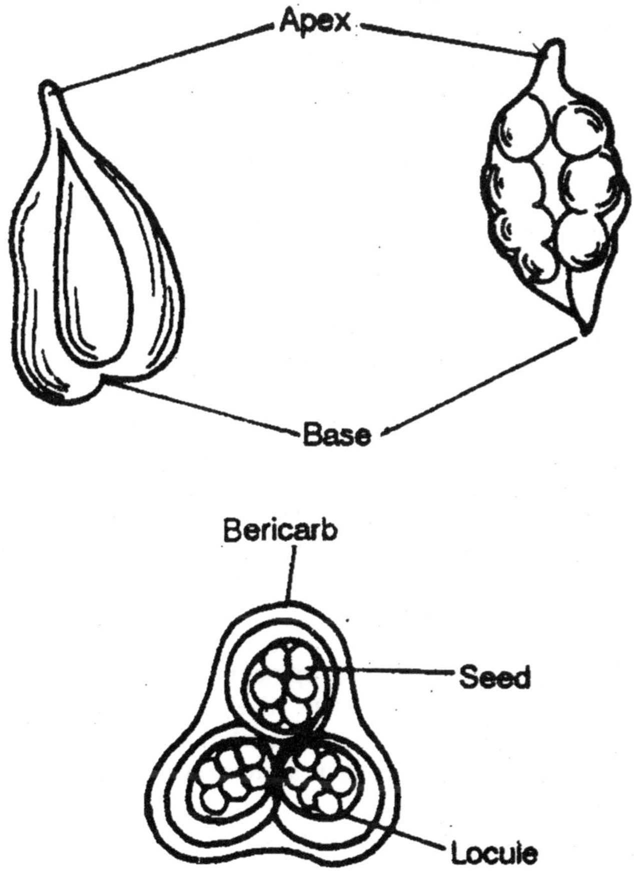

Carrier

One who harbours a disease organism but does not have the symptoms.

2. A person who has a recessive mutated gene, together with its normal allele. Carriers do not usually develop disease but can pass the mutated gene on to their children.

Cascara Sagrada (Rhamnus purshiana)

The bark a gentle laxative26 especially helpful for the elderly27, particularly in cases of chronic constipation; antispasmodic; and strengthens the liver28; a chelating agent to prevent the formation of calcium-containing urinary stones; used for hepatic **disease29. contraindicated during pregnancy.**

Catabolism

The intracellular phase of metabolism involved in the energy-yielding degradation of nutrient molecules (for example, glucose to CO_2 and H_2O). Waste products are called catabolites.

Catalase

An enzyme that catalyzes the decomposition of hydrogen peroxide and molecular oxygen and water.

Catalyst

A compound that increases the rate of a chemical reaction without being consumed or changed. In the biosciences, the term enzyme is used. Enzymes catalyze biological reactions.

Catecholamine

Biologically active amines, epinephrine, norepinephrine, and dopamine derived from the amino acid tyrosine. Catecholamines function as neurotransmitters and hormones in the brain, cardiovascular system, and smooth muscle.

Cat's Claw (Uncaria tomentosa)

Detoxifier.

Cation

A positively charged particle or ion.

Cation Exchange

The displacement of one positively charged particle by another on a cation-exchange material.

Cation Exchange Resin

An Ion exchange resin, which removes positively charged ions (cations) by exchanging them for hydrogen ions.

Catnip (Nepeta cataria)

Associated with stomach discomforts30; carminative (an agent use to relieve gas and sharp pain in the bowel region); antispasmodic; relieves cold and flu symptoms; a diaphoretic; a mild antimicrobial. (North American Indians used catnip tea for colic in babies). contraindicated during **pregnancy.**

Cavitation

A condition of liquid flow where, after partial vaporization of the liquid, the subsequent collapse of vapor bubbles can produce surface damage.

Cayenne (Capsicum annum)

A blood purifier; lowers blood cholesterol levels; helps reduce blood pressure24; improves circulation and respiration25.

CBER

(also see: center for Biologics Evaluation and Research)

Celery

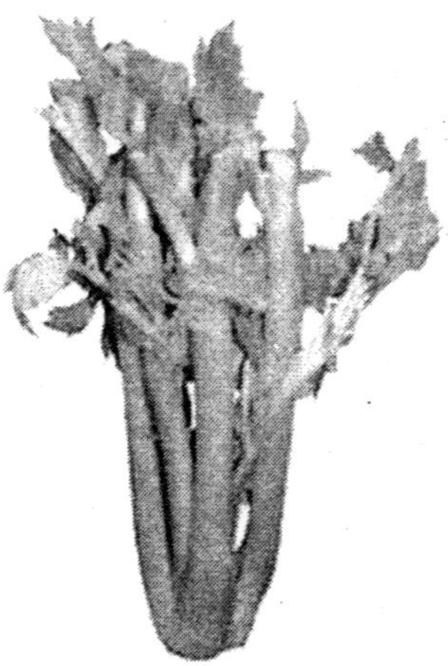

Apium graveolens

Celery *(Apium graveolens L.)* is a vegetable, more specifically a biennial plant belonging to the order Umbelliferae (Apiales). It has a furrowed stalk with wedge-shaped leaves, the whole plant having a coarse, rank taste, and a peculiar smell. With cultivation and blanching, the stalks lose their acrid qualities and assume the mild, sweetish, aromatic taste peculiar to celery as a salad plant.

The plants are raised from seed, sown either in a hot bed or in the open garden according to the season of the year, and after one or two thinnings out and transplantings they are, on attaining a height of 6 or 8 inches, planted out in deep trenches for convenience of blanching, which is effected by earthing up, and so excluding stems from the influence of light.

A large number of varieties are cultivated by gardeners, which are ranged under two classes, white and red - the white varieties being generally the best flavoured, and most crisp and tender.

In the past, celery was grown as a vegetable for winter and early spring; because of its antitoxic properties, it was a cleansing tonic after the stagnation of winter.

In its native condition, it is known in England as smallage. In its wild state, it is common by the sides of ditches and in marshy places, especially near the sea.

Celeriac is a variety of celery, *Apium graveolens* var. *rapaceum*, cultivated for its roots rather than its stalks, although both are edible and are used for salads and in soups. It is chiefly grown in the north of Europe.

Celery seed is used as a spice. The homeopathic extract of the seeds is widely used in France to relieve retention of urine.

- As a salad plant, celery, especially if at all "stringy", is difficult to digest but possesses valuable diuretic properties.
- Both blanched and green it is stewed and used soups, the seeds also being used as a flavouring ingredient. Even after long immersion in broth, the stalks remain somewhat crisp, and useful for adding texture to the soup.
- In the south of Europe celery is seldom blanched, but is much used in its natural condition.
- Chopped, it is one of the three vegetables considered the holy trinity of Louisiana Creole and Cajun cuisine.

The whole plant is gently stimulant, nourishing, and restorative; it can be liquefied, with the juice taken for joint and urinary tract inflammations, such as rheumatoid arthritis, cystitis, or urethritis, for weak conditions, and for nervous exhaustion.

More specific uses:

- **Seeds** Mainly used as a diuretic, these help clear toxins from the system, so are especially good for gout, where uric acid crystals collect in the joints, and arthritis. Slightly bitter, they act as a mild digestive stimulant. Harvest after the plant flowers in its second year. Infuse the seeds for rheumatoid arthritis and gout, combine 2 tsp. lignum vitae, and add 1/2 tsp. to a cup of boiling water.
- **Essential oil** Distilled from the seeds, the essential oil is more potent therapeutically. Use with care. 'Oil' can be used for painful gout in the feet or toes, add 15 drops oil to a bowl of warm water, and soak the feet. 'Massage oil' can be made by diluting 5-10 drops celery oil in 20 ml almond or sunflower oil, and massage into arthritic joints.
- **Root** Rarely used today, the root is an effective diuretic and has been taken for urinary stones and gravel. It also acts as a bitter digestive remedy and liver stimulant. A tincture can be used as a diuretic in hypertension and urinary disorders, as a component in arthritic remedies, or as a kidney energy stimulant and cleanser.
- Bergapten in the seeds could increase photosensitivity, so do not apply the essential oil externally in bright sunshine.
- Avoid the oil and large doses of the seeds during pregnancy: they can act as a uterine stimulant.
- Do not buy seeds intended for cultivation, because they are often treated with fungicides.

There is a widespread myth that the word celery (*The Fast Vegetable)* has roots in the Latin word, *celer*, meaning fast or swift. This is entirely false - there is no connection between them. It actually comes from the Greek selinon, meaning parsley. It passed through Latin, Italian and French before becoming the modern English word celery.

Celsius

Of or pertaining to a temperature scale that registers the

freezing point of water as 0°C and the boiling point as 100°C under normal atmospheric pressure. Also called "centigrade". The designation Celsius has been official since 1948, but centigrade remains in common use.

Cell

The fundamental unit of life. The living tissue of almost every organism is composed of these fundamental living units. Unicellular organisms, such as yeast or a bacterium, perform all life functions within the one cell. In a higher organism, a multicellular organism, entire populations of cells may be designated a particular task. The cells of muscle tissue, for example, are specialized for movement.

Cell Bank

Master Cell Bank: The bank of cells, which contain the original unused mutated cells from which, the Manufacturing Working Cell Bank is taken. This is usually kept under lock with very limited access.

Manufacturing Working Cell Bank: The bank of cells derived from the Master Cell Bank, which are used to seed the fermentation manufacturing process.

Cell Culture

The in vitro propagation of cells removed from organisms in a laboratory environment that has strict sterility, temperature, and nutrient requirement; also used to refer to any particular individual sample. Usually, cell culture takes place in a bioreactor.

Cell Differentiation

The process whereby descendants of a common parental cell achieve and maintain specialization of structure and function. Muscle cells become muscle cells and bone cells develop. In humans all the different types of cells differentiate from the simple sperm and egg.

Cell Fusion

The fusing together of two or more cells to become a single cell. This technique has had important consequences in immunology, developmental biology, and genetics. For example, monoclonal antibodies are produced by fusing a spleen cell (producing an antibody specific for the antigen of interest) with a mouse myeloma cell to produce a hybridoma which has an indefinitely long life because of the myeloma component and which secretes a specific antibody. When a human cell is fused with a mouse cell, the human chromosomes are progressively lost from the resultant hybrid and by correlating the presence of proteins in the hybrid with the presence of particular human chromosomes, genes can be assigned to individual chromosomes.

Cell Lines

When cells from the first culture (taken from the organism) are used to make subsequent cultures, a cell line is established. "Immortal" cell lines can replicate indefinitely.

Cellulose

A polymer of six-carbon sugars found in all plant matter, the most abundant biological compound on earth.

Center For Biologics Evaluation and Research (CBER)

The FDA successor to the Bureau of Biologics concerned with biologic drugs, and most importantly, with the new protein and peptide drugs emanating from biotechnology.

Center For Drug Evaluation and Research (CDER)

The successor to the Bureau of Drugs of the FDA concerned with all SVPs (Small Volume Parenterals), LVPs (Large Volume Parenterals), and non-biological drugs.

Centimorgan (cM)

A unit of measure of recombination frequency. One centimorgan is equal to a 1% chance that a marker at one genetic locus will be separated from a marker at a second locus due to crossing over in a single generation. In human beings, one centimorgan is equivalent, on average, to one million base pairs.

Centrifugation

Mechanical means of separation based on differences in sedimentation rates due to differences in density between the suspended particles in the liquid.

Centrifuge

A centrifuge operates on the principle of centrifugal force, the inertial reaction by which a body tends to move away from a center about which it revolves. This technique is commonly used to separate solids from liquids or liquids of different densities. Centrifugal equipment is divided into two major types, sedimenters and filters:

Sedimenters

For sedimentation, batch and continuous centrifuges are available. There are three types of centrifuges for continuous sedimentation.

a) Disc - constructed on the vertical axis, disc centrifuges are solid-bowl units. All are capable of separating liquids from solids, solids from two immiscible liquids and two immiscible liquids. Disc-stack centrifuges differ in their ability to handle different volumes of solids in the feed stream, and in the way that the separated solids are removed from the separation vessel: solids-retaining, solids-ejecting, and nozzle-bowl separators.

b) Decanters - consists of a cylindrical settling section with a tapered end. Inside the bowl is a scroll conveyor that is driven usually at a slightly faster rate than the bowl and can be controlled by a differential speed device or back drive.

c) Tubular - a vertical solid-wall cylinder provided with caps on both ends; a tubular centrifuge generally has a bottom feed inlet. When two liquids of different specific gravities are fed, the heavier phase is concentrated against the wall, while the lighter phase "floats" on the heavier phase.

Filters

Filtering centrifuges accommodate a range of liquid-solid separations. The two batch types, basket and peeler centrifuges, can separate almost any liquid-solid slurry. For continuous operation, there are pusher and conical centrifuges.

a) Pusher - with a horizontal axis, the pusher centrifuge operates at a constant fixed speed. It has a perforated bowl,

generally with a bar-type screen. One end of the bowl is open while the opposite end is closed with a reciprocating diaphragm, or disc, which rotates with the bowl.
b) Conical - the standard conical centrifuge consists of a cone with a small closed end and a large open end to which is attached a coarsely woven drainage screen, topped with a filter screen or perforated plate. A compartmentalized casing surrounds the bowl. There are two variations of the basic conical centrifuge: the tilting conical centrifuge and the conveyor conical type.

Centromere
A specialized chromosome region to which mitotic or meiotic spindle fibers attach during cell division.

Cerebroprotective
A substance or procedure that protects brain cells from ischemic damage due to hypoxia, as in cerebral aneurysms.

Certification
Documented testimony by qualified authorities that a system qualification, calibration, validation, or revalidation has been performed appropriately and that the results are acceptable. Personnel certification is proof that a person has achieved a certain level of qualification.

Certified Vendor Drawings
Drawings prepared by vendors for the fabrication of equipment, specialty components and skid mounted systems. These are certified as fabricated by the vendor and become the official document for the equipment involved.

CFR (Code of Federal regulations) Title 21
The U.S. regulations that directly apply to biopharmaceutical development are contained in Title 21 parts 58 (Good Laboratory Practice for Nonclinical Laboratory Studies), 210 (Current Good Manufacturing Practice in Manufacturing, Processing, Packing, or Holding of Drugs; General), 211 (Current Good Manufacturing Practice for Finished Pharmaceuticals), and 600 (Biological Products: General).

Parts 50 (Protection of Human Subjects), 56 (Institutional Review Boards), and 312 (Investigational New Drugs) apply to critical trials.

Part 11 provides criteria which will consider electronic records to be equivalent to paper records and electronic signatures to be equivalent to traditional handwritten signatures. (also see: cGMPs (current Good Manufacturing Practices)).

CFU (Colony Forming Unit)

A measure of the number of bacteria present in the environment or on the surfaces of an aseptic processing room, measured as part of qualification and ongoing monitoring. Also applied to the testing of purified water samples.

cGMPs (current Good Manufacturing Practices)

Current accepted standards of design, operation, practice, and sanitization. The FDA is empowered to inspect drug-manufacturing plants in which drugs are processed, manufactured, packaged, and stored for compliance with these standards.

Chamomile (Matricaria chamomilla)

The flowers reduce stomach problems, helps relieve cancer of the liver, mouth, skin and brain, applied internally as well as externally31; calms anxiety; stimulates the expulsion of parasitic worms in the digestive system; also helps eliminate of bacteria that cause strep throat32; used to treat skin problems33. The essential oil's in Chamomile are a wonderful blend of many individual oils. Pharmacological research suggested that there is a strengthening the protective mucosal barrier against ulceration. Action: Nervine, anti-spasmodic, carminative, anti-inflammatory, anti-microbial, bitter,and vulnerary.

Change Control

A formal system by which qualified representatives of appropriate disciplines review proposed or actual changes that might affect a validated process's status. The intent is to determine the need for action that would ensure that the system is maintained in a validated state.

Change Over

The program by which a processing area is cleared of supplies and components used in the manufacture of a previous product and then readied for production of a new product. This often includes parts change over and/or special cleaning to eliminate cross-contamination.

Channeling

Cleavage, cracking, and furrowing of a resin bed due to resin age, a change in one of the feed solutions, or faulty operational procedures. The solution being treated follows the path of least resistance, runs through these furrows, and fails to contact active resin material in other parts of the bed.

Characterization

Precisely deciphering and describing all the characteristics of a drug substance that affect its efficacy and its purity. Or the chemical, physical, and sometimes biological properties that are attributes of a specific drug substance.

Checksum

A record of the number of bits transmitted and included with the transmission so that the receiving program can check to see whether the same number of bits arrived. If the counts match, it is assumed that the complete transmission was received.

Chelating Agents

Organic compounds that can withdraw ions from solution, forming insoluble complexes.

Chemoautotrophs

Facultative autotrophs that obtain their energy from the oxidation of inorganic compounds.

Chemostat

A growth chamber that keeps a bacterial culture at a specific volume and rate of growth by limiting nutrient medium and removing spent culture.

Chemotherapy

The use of a drug, or combination of drugs, to kill or inhibit the growth of microorganisms or cancer.

2. Treatment of disease by means of chemical substances or drugs.

Chestnut (Castanea Sativa)

Contracts body tissue and blood vessels; helps in convulsive coughs and other irritable conditions of the respiratory organs.

Chickweed (Stellaria media)

Reduces internal inflammation, and external swelling; soothes coughs, colds, sore throats, and flus34; effective against certain respiratory pathogens35.

Chicory

Chicory is a flowering plant in genus Cichorium in family Asteraceae. There are two important species in genus Cichorium.

Chicory (Cichorium intybus) is a perennial herb with flowers that are usually blue. It is originally from the Old World and was naturalized in North America, where it is seen as a rank, roadside weed. At times, its roots have been used as a substitute for coffee. It is also used as a flavoring in coffee.

Endive (*Cichorium endivia*) is a popular salad green, having a slightly bitter taste. It has also been attributed with herbal properties. Endive is often confused with chicory.

There are three principal types of endive: Belgian endive, curly endive and escarole:

Belgian endive (also known as French endive or witloof) has a small head of cream-coloured bitter leaves. It is grown in complete darkness to avoid the leaves turning green.

Curly endive (sometimes mistakenly called chicory in the United States) has green rimmed curly outer leaves.

Escarole has broad, pale green leaves and is less bitter than the other varieties.

Dig beside the chicory root with a long tool and cut it down deep. (Don't pull the leaves. They tear off more easily than the root pulls out.) Cut off the leaves and peel the roots. Split the roots and wash them because they may have soil inside. Next, cut the roots into long strips. Bake them at 140C (250F) for four hours. Maybe a little higher. Last, grind as you would coffee and add into coffee one for one...or boil only the ground chicory (one spoon per cup) for three minutes instead of coffee.

Chile (capsicum)

The chile pepper (also chili or chilli; from Nahuatl chilli via Spanish chile) is the fruit of the plant Capsicum from the nightshade family (Solanaceae).

The chile peppers and their various cultivars are grown around the world because they are widely used as spices or vegetables in cuisine, and even as medicine.

Cultivated since prehistoric times in Peru and Mexico, it was discovered in the Caribbean by Columbus and named a "pepper" because of its similarity with the Old World peppers of the Piper *genus.*

Diego Alvarez Chanca, a physician on Columbus' second voyage to the West Indies in 1493, brought the first chile peppers to Spain, and first wrote about their medicinal effects in 1494.

The most common species of chile peppers are:

- Capsicum annuum, which includes many common varieties such as bell peppers, paprika, and jalapeños
- Capsicum frutescens, which includes the cayenne and tabasco peppers
- Capsicum chinense, which includes the hottest peppers such as habaneros and Scotch bonnets
- Capsicum pubescens, which includes the South American rocoto peppers
- Capsicum baccatum, which includes the chiltepin

Though there are only a few commonly used species, there are many cultivars and methods of preparing chile peppers that have different common names for culinary use. Green and red bell peppers, for example, are the same cultivar of C. annuum, *the green ones being immature. In the same species are the jalapeño, the chipotle (a smoked jalapeño), the poblano, ancho (which is a dried poblano), New Mexico, Anaheim, Serrano, and other cultivars. Jamaicans, Scotch bonnets, and habaneros are common varieties of*

C. chinense. *The species* C. frutescens *appears as chiles de arbol, aji, pequin, tabasco, cayenne, cherry peppers, and others.*

Heat

The substances that give chiles their heat are the alkaloid capsaicin (8-methyl-N-vanillyl-6-nonenamide) and four related chemicals, collectively called capsaicinoids. Each capsaicinoid has a different effect on the mouth, and variation in the proportions of these chemical is responsible for the differing sensations produced by different varieties. Capsaicin causes pain and inflammation if consumed to excess, and can even burn the skin on contact in high concentrations (habanero peppers, for example, are routinely picked with gloves). It is also the primary ingredient in pepper spray, which is used as a "less-than-lethal" weapon.

The "heat" of chile peppers is measured in Scoville units. Bell peppers rank at zero Scoville units, jalapeños at 3,000–6,000 Scoville units, and habaneros at 300,000 Scoville units. The record for the highest number of Scoville units in a pepper is assigned by the Guinness Book of Records to the Red Savina Habanero, measuring 577,000 units. However, a recent report was made of a pepper from India called the Naga Jolokia measuring at 855,000 Scoville units. Both the Red Savina and the Naga Jolokia claims are disputed as to their validity, and lack independent verification. Pure capsaicin rates at 16,000,000 Scoville units.

Chimeric

An organism, especially a plant, containing tissues from at least two genetically distinct parents. Type of antibody, partially human and partially mouse.

Chloramine

A chlorine compound formed by reaction with organic amines or ammonia.

Chlorinated Vinyls

Thermoplastic chlorinated vinyls include PVC, CPVC, and VDC. PVC and CPVC are very similar materials, the primary difference being the addition of more chlorine to the PVC molecule to synthesize CPVC. This results in a higher glass transition temperature that equates to a higher use temperature for CPVC. The polymerization with chlorine also makes these materials inherently flame resistant. In addition to being resistant to higher temperatures, CPVC is more resistant to process chemicals.

Chlorination

Adding chlorine or chlorine compounds to water for disinfection.

Chlorine

An element used to kill microorganisms in water. At room temperature and atmospheric pressure a greenish yellow gas.

Chlorine Demand

Amount of chlorine used up by reacting with oxidizable substances in water before chlorine residual can be measured.

Chlorine Residual

Portion of free or combined chlorine that remains active after specified contact period.

Chloroplasts

Relatively large, chlorophyll containing, green organelles responsible for photosynthesis in photosynthetic eukaryotes, such as algae and plant cells. Every chloroplast contains an outer membrane and a large number of inner membranes called thylakoids.

CHO (Chinese Hamster Ovary) Cells

In cell culture, the cells of a female hamster's reproductive organs, which historically have proven to be excellent expression systems in analytical studies and for producing pharmaceutical proteins.

Cholesterol

A sterol widely distributed in animal tissues and occurring in egg yolks, fats, nerve tissue, the liver, kidneys, and adrenal glands. It is the precursor of various steroid hormones and is a normal constituent of bile.

Chromatids

Copies of a chromosome produced by replication.

Chromatin

The complex of DNA and protein in the nucleus of the interphase cell, originally recognized by its reaction with stains specific for DNA..

Chromatography

This word applies to various different methods of chemical analysis that separate and detect compounds or groups of compounds from a complex mixture. Types of chromatography include TLC (thin layer chromatography), HPTLC (high performance thin layer chromatography), HPLC (high performance liquid chromatography), GC (gas chromatography - or GC/MS: gas chromatography/mass spectrometry), and GLC (gas liquid chromatography). The word is made up of Greek roots meaning 'color' and 'writing,' because early chromatographs separated colored compounds into bands on a flat surface.

2. Procedure by which solutes (e.g., proteins and other chemical products) are selectively separated by a dynamic differential migration process in a system consisting of two or more phases, one of which moves continuously in a given direction and in which the individual substances exhibit different mobilities by reason of differences in adsorption, partition, solubility, vapor pressure, molecular size, or ionic charge density. The individual substances thus obtained can be identified or determined by analytical methods. There are several types of chromatography in use with different operating principles:

1. Adsorption - separates products by their different affinities for the surface of a solid medium, either an inorganic carrier such as silica gel, alumina, or hydroxyapatite, or an organic polymer.

2. Ion Exchange - uses ion exchange resin to which ionized functional groups have been attached. At an appropriate pH, target proteins acquire a net surface charge that allows them to selectively bind to an ion exchange resin. Other impurities are eluted through the column.

3. Gel Filtration - employs a neutral cross-linked carrier with

a defined pore size for molecular fractionation. Molecules larger than the largest pores cannot enter the matrix and pass directly through the column; smaller molecules enter the carrier and are retarded. Gel filtration thus separates on the basis of molecular size, eluting larger molecules first, followed by progressively smaller species.

4. Affinity - relies on the propensity of each biomolecule to have an affinity for another highly specific biomolecule, such as an antibody-antigen relationship. Once bound together, the drug molecules can be detached by altering various chemical attributes in the column.

5. Hydrophobic - separates by molecule polarity and reverse interaction with water.

6. High Pressure Liquid Chromatography (HPLC)- Various methods of separating individual chemical constituents out of complex mixtures.

Chromium Enrichment Layer Thickness

In stainless steel, the same as its maximum depth of enrichment, unless a surface iron layer is present in which case the chromium enrichment layer is calculated as the maximum depth of enrichment minus the thickness of the surface iron oxide layer.

Chromosome

The self-replicating genetic structure of cells containing the cellular DNA that bears in its nucleotide sequence the linear array of genes. In prokaryotes, chromosomal DNA is circular, and the entire genome is carried on one chromosome. Eukaryotic genomes consist of a number of chromosomes whose DNA is associated with different kind of proteins.

Chronic effect

Adverse effects in which symptoms develop slowly over a period of time and with multiple low doses.

Cinchona

Cinchona is the dried bark of *Cinchona calisays, C. ledgeriana, C. officinalis* and *C. Succirubra.*

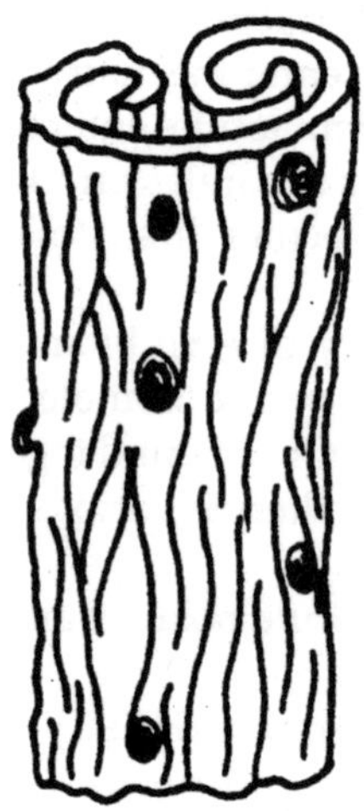

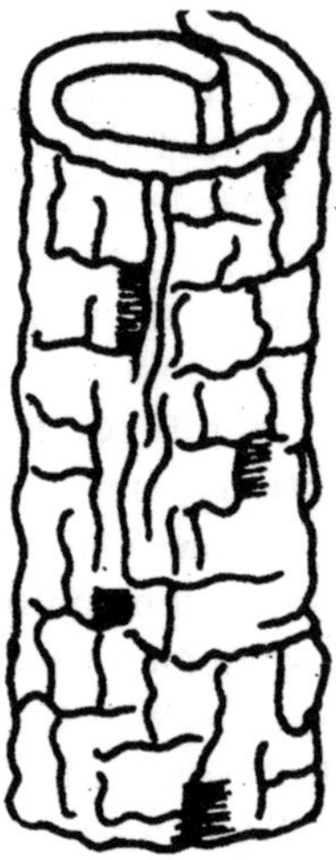

Cinamon

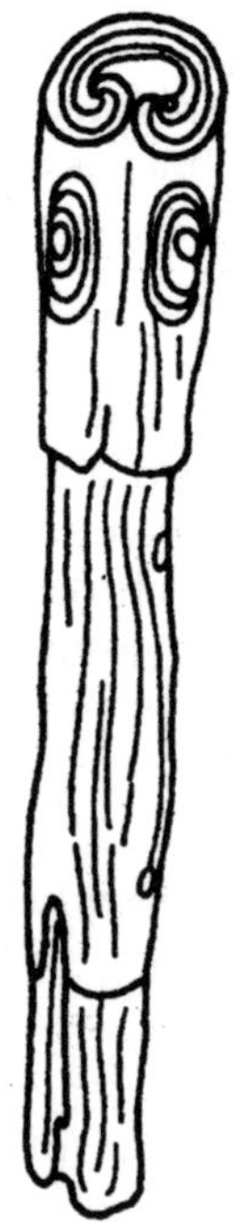

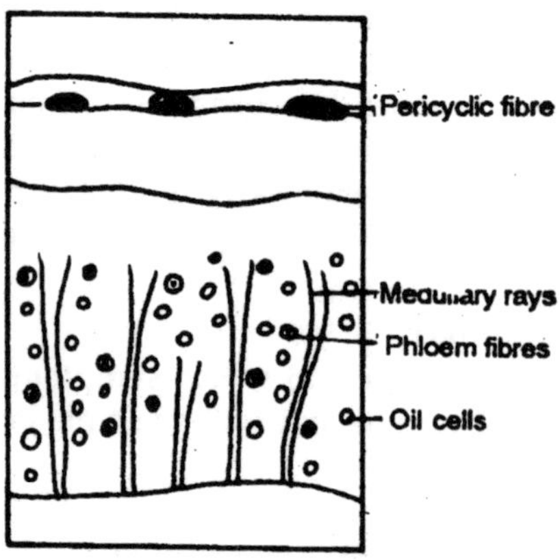

Cinnamon Bark

The drug consists of the bark obtained from *Cinnamomum zeylanicum*.

CIP (Clean In Place)

Internally cleaning a piece of equipment without relocation or disassembly. The equipment is cleaned but not necessarily sterilized. The cleaning is normally done by acid, caustic, or a combination of both, with WFI rinse. The design of a CIP system should considered the operating volume design for the water consumption, chemical and biowaste effluent, and energy required to clean a given circuit or piece of equipment.

Class 100

Classification of an aseptic processing area where particle count should not exceed 100 particles (3,530 particles per cubic meter) 0.5µm or larger, per cubic foot of air, and no more than 0.1 CFU (Colony Forming Units) per cubic foot. Target uniform air velocity is 90 fpm plus or minus 20%, HEPA filtered air. (also see Table I, Section II - Comparison of Airborne Particulate Cleanliness Classes)

Class 1,000

Classification of an area where particle count should not exceed 1,000 particles (35,300 particles per cubic meter) 0.5µm or larger, per cubic foot of air. Supplied by HEPA filtered air. Class 1,000 is not a pharmaceutical GMP expectation. (also see Table I, Section II - Comparison of Airborne Particulate Cleanliness Classes)

Class 10,000

Classification of an area where particle count should not exceed 10,000 particles (353,000 particles per cubic meter) 0.5µm or larger, per cubic foot of air. Minimum of 20 air changes per hour, HEPA filtered air. (also see Table I, Section II - Comparison of Airborne Particulate Cleanliness Classes)

Class 100,000

Classification of an area where particle count should not exceed 100,000 particles (3,530,000 particles per cubic meter) 0.5µm or larger, per cubic foot of air, and no more than 2.5

CFU (Colony Forming Units) per cubic foot. Minimum of 20 air changes per hour of HEPA filtered air. (also see Table I, Section II - Comparison of Airborne Particulate Cleanliness Classes)

Class Name

"For naming and describing the classes, SI names and units are preferred; however, English (U.S. customary) units may be used". Federal Standard 209E superseded by ISO 14644-1). (also see Table I, Section II - Comparison of Airborne Particulate Cleanliness Classes)

Class 95% ASHRAE Area

This area designation refers to the efficiency of the filters based on ASHRAE standard 52-76. These areas would have 95% efficient supply air filtration, unlike classified areas, which would have HEPA filtration. This classification is not specified in Federal Standard 209E or ISO 14644-1.

Class 65% ASHRAE Area

This area would have 65% efficient filtration. This classification is not specified in Federal Standard 209E or ISO 14644-1.

Class 30% ASHRAE Area

This area would have 30% efficient filtration. This classification is not specified in Federal Standard 209E or ISO 14644-1.

Classical Pharmaceuticals

Small-molecule, nonbiotech drugs produced by chemical synthesis.

Classification

The level (or the process of specifying or determining the level) of airborne particulate cleanliness applicable to a cleanroom or clean zone, expressed in terms of an ISO Class N, which represents maximum allowable concentrations (in particles per cubic meter of air) for considered sizes of particles. ISO 14644-1 (also see Table I, Section II - Comparison of Airborne Particulate Cleanliness Classes)

Classified Space

A space in which the number of airborne particles is limited. This is accomplished by the strict use of HVAC systems. Areas are classified as Class 10, Class 100, Class 1,000, Class 10,000, and Class 100,000. In pharmaceutical production, only classes 100, 10,000, and 100,000 are used. (also see Table I, Section II - Comparison of Airborne Particulate Cleanliness Classes).

Clean Air Projector

Fan and filter unit used to locally clean room air and deliver it to a desired location. Often called a fan/filter unit.

Clean Area

An area where particulate and microbial levels are specified (e.g., Filling Room - Class 10,000 "In Operation")

Clean In Place (CIP)

(also see: CIP (Clean In Place))

Cleanroom

A specially constructed space environmentally controlled with respect to airborne particles (size and count), temperature, humidity, air pressure, airflow patterns, air motion, and lighting. ISO 14644-1 defines it as "a room in which the concentration of airborne particles is controlled, and which is constructed and used in a manner to minimize the introduction, generation, and retention of particles inside the room, and in which other relevant parameters, e.g. temperature, humidity, and pressure, are controlled as necessary." (also see Table I, Section II - Comparison of Airborne Particulate Cleanliness Classes)

Cleanroom Classification

The maximum number of particles greater than or equal to 0.5µm in diameter that may be present in a cubic foot of room air.

Clean Space

A room or volume controlled to meet a certain airborne particulate limit (Class or Grade). In pharmaceutical facilities, clean spaces are usually classified and controlled only for aseptic processing facilities, but may also be defined for certain biotech processes. Final non-sterile bulk facilities, oral product, most topical product manufacturing facilities, and warehouses are normally not classified as clean spaces.

Clean Steam

Steam free from boiler additives that may be purified, filtered, or separated. When condensed, clean steam meets the specification for WFI. Usually utilized to sterilize process equipment.

Clean Zone

ISO 14644-1 defines it as "a dedicated space in which the concentration of airborne particles is controlled, and which is constructed and used in a manner to minimize the introduction, generation, and retention of particles inside the zone and in which other relevant parameters, e.g. temperature, humidity, and pressure, are controlled as necessary". Additionally, ISO 14644-1 states, "this zone may be open or enclosed and may or may not be located within a cleanroom".

Cleavage

The splitting up of a complex molecule into two or more simpler molecules. The series of cell divisions occurring in the ovum immediately following its fertilization.

Climate change

Refers to the consequences of the buildup of anthropogenic gases in the atmosphere which trap the sun's heat, causing changes in the weather pattern on a global scale.

Climax Community

The relative stable community reached by a successional series.

Clinical Endpoint

An indicator (such as blood pressure) measured in a human subject to asses the safety, efficacy, or other objective of a clinical trial.

Coenzyme A

Enzyme important in a variety of biological processes, including sterol and fatty acid synthesis, and in energy metabolism.

Colchcium

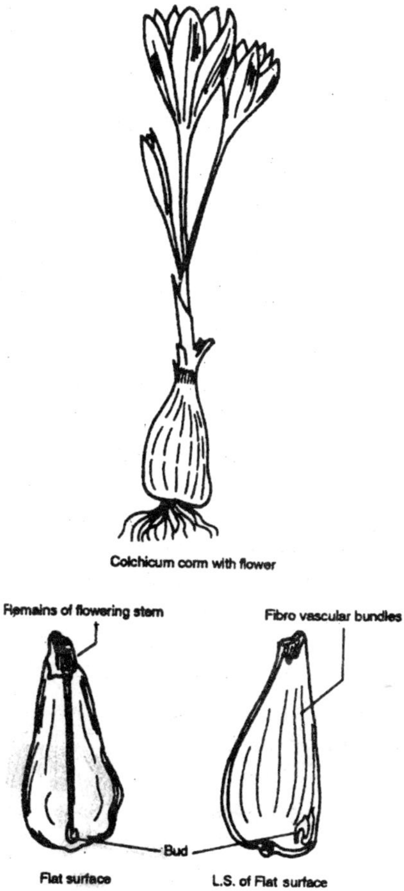

Colchcium

The drug consists of seeds and corms of *Colchicum autumbale* Linn. India drug is obtained from *Colchicum luteum* Baker.

Coriander

Coriander is the dried ripe fruit obtained from *Coriandrum sativum.*

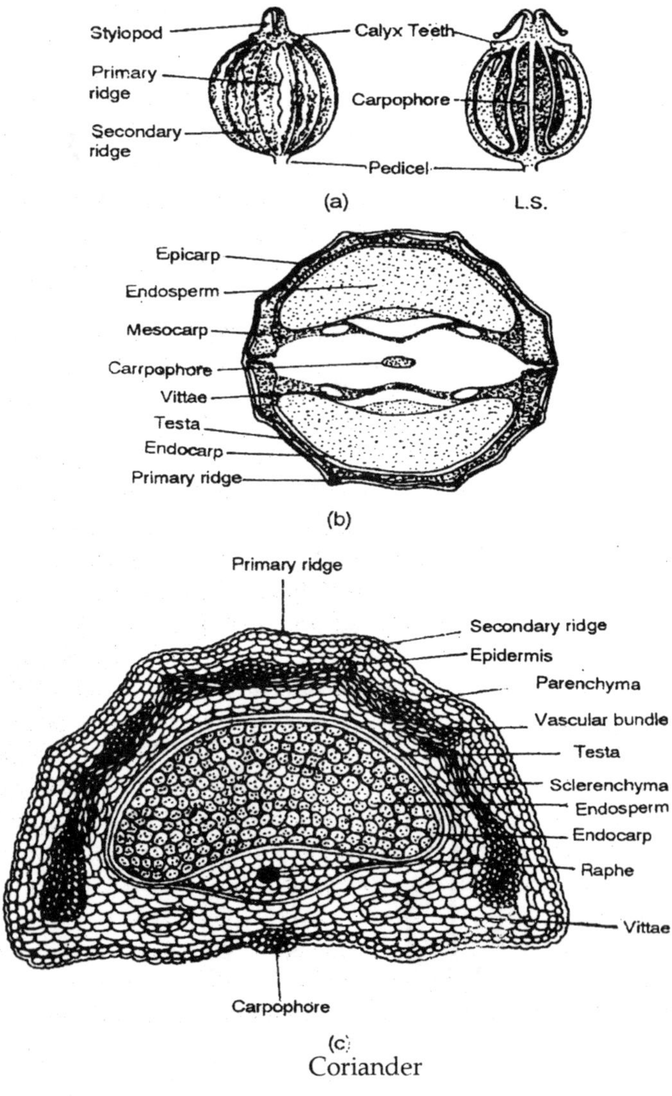

Coriander

Collagen

A fibrous insoluble protein found in connective tissue, including skin, bone, ligaments, and cartilage.

Community

All the organisms of a given taxonomic rank (ie animal, plant, microbial community). Also applied to geographical regions (biomes) as in a tundra community or salt marsh community.

Compound

A chemical composed of more than one type of atom. For example, Sulfur (S) is an element, but allicin is a compound containing sulfur, oxygen, carbon and hydrogen.

Contraindication

Any symptom or circumstance indicating the inappropriateness of a treatment otherwise advisable.

Cotton

Cotton is the epidermal hairs of the seeds of cultivated species of *Gossypium herbaceum*.

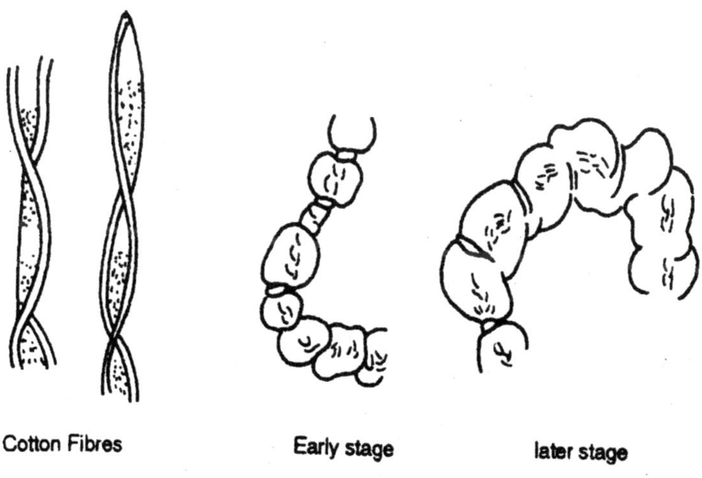

Cotton Fibres — Early stage — later stage

Cotton Fibres

Coumarins

A class of chemical compounds, widespread in plants, which contain a coumarinic acid lactone.

Crossover study

Experimental design protocol in which the control group and the treated group are exchanged in the second phase of the study.

Cuisine

The fruit is eaten cooked or raw for its fiery hot flavor which is concentrated along the top of the pod. The stem end of the pod has glands which produce the capsaicin, which then flows down through the pod. Removing the seeds and inner membranes is thus effective at reducing the heat of a pod.

Well-known dishes with a strong chile flavor are Mexican salsas, Tex-Mex chili con carne, and Indian vindaloos and other curries. Chili powder is a spice made of the dried ground chiles, usually of the Mexican chile ancho variety, but with small amounts of cayenne added for heat. Bottled hot sauces such as Tabasco sauce are made from chiles such as the cayenne (not, oddly, from tabasco peppers), which may also be fermented.

Indian, Szechuan and Thai cuisines are particularly associated with the chile pepper, although the plant was unknown in Asia until Europeans introduced it there.

Chile peppers are popular in food, despite the pain and irritation they bring. Capsaicin has an antibacterial effect, so food cooked with chiles keeps for longer without spoiling. Chiles are rich in vitamin C and are believed to have many beneficial effects on health. The pain caused by capsaicin stimulates the brain to produce endorphins, natural opioids which act as analgesics and produce a sense of well-being. Psychologist Paul Rozin suggests that eating chiles is an example of a "constrained risk" like riding a roller coaster, in which extreme sensations like pain and fear can be enjoyed because we know they are not actually harmful.

Birds do not have the same sensitivity to capsaicin as mammals, as capsaicin acts on a specific nerve receptor in mammals, and avian nervous systems are rather different.

Chile peppers are in fact a favorite food of many birds living in the chile peppers' natural range. The flesh of the peppers provides the birds with nutritious meal rich in vitamin C. In return, the seeds of the peppers are distributed by the birds, as they drop the seeds while eating the pods or the seeds pass through the digestive tract unharmed. This relationship is theorized to have promoted the evolution of the protective capsaicin. It is interesting to note that the chemical used to give an artificial grape flavoring to food items such as grape soda does have a similar effect on birds as capsaicin has on humans.

- Chile is the most common spelling which refers specifically to this plant and its fruit. This orthography is universal in the Spanish-speaking world, even though in some parts chile is better known as ají.
- Chili is also quite popular, but its use is discouraged by some, as this word is more commonly used to refer to a popular Southwestern dish (chili is the official state dish of Texas[2] (http://www.tsl.state.tx.us/ref/abouttx/symbols/chili.html)), as well as to the mixture of cumin and other spices (chili powder) used to flavor it.
- The alternative spelling chilli is used in non-American English speaking countries such as the UK and Australia.
- The name of this plant bears no relation to Chile, the country, which is named after the Quechua chin (cold), tchili (snow), or chilli (where the land ends).

Cinnamon

Cinnamon (Cinnamomum zeylanicum, *synonym* C. verum*) is* a small evergreen tree 10-15 m tall, belonging to the family

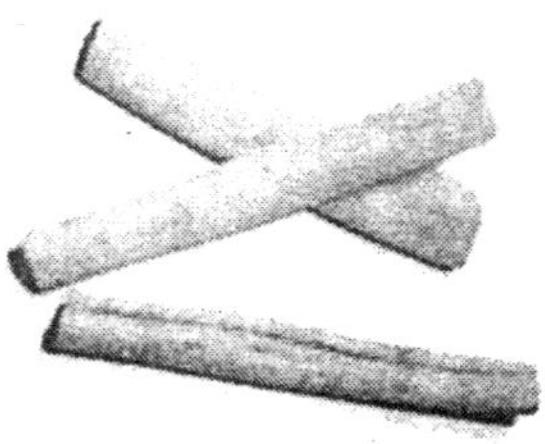

Sticks of cinnamon bark

Lauraceae, and a spice obtained from the inner bark of this species. It is native to Sri Lanka. The leaves are ovate-oblong in shape, 7-18 cm long. The flowers, which are arranged in panicles, have a greenish colour and a rather disagreeable odour. The fruit is a purple 1 cm berry containing a single seed.

Cinnamon is principally employed in cookery as a condiment and flavouring material, being largely used in the preparation of some kinds of chocolate and liqueurs. In medicine it acts like other volatile oils and once had a reputation as a "cure" for colds. The pungent taste and scent come from cinnamic aldehyde or cinnamaldehyde.

The best cinnamon is from Sri Lanka, but the tree is also grown at Tellicherry in Java, Sumatra, the West Indies, Brazil, Madagascar, and Egypt. Sri Lanka cinnamon of fine quality is a very thin smooth bark, with a light-yellowish brown colour, a highly fragrant odour, and a peculiarly sweet, warm and pleasing aromatic taste. Its flavour is due to an aromatic oil which it contains to the extent of from 0.5 to 1%. This essential oil, as an article of commerce, is prepared by roughly pounding the bark, macerating it in sea-water, and then quickly distilling the whole. It is of a golden-yellow colour, with the peculiar odour of cinnamon and a very hot aromatic taste. It consists essentially of cinnamic aldehyde and, by the absorption of oxygen as it ages, it darkens in colour and develops resinous compounds.

Cinnamon has been known from remote antiquity, and it was so highly prized among ancient nations that it was regarded as a present fit for monarchs and other great potentates. It is mentioned in Exodus 30: 23, where Moses is commanded to use both sweet cinnamon (Kinnamon) and cassia, and in Proverbs 7: 17-18, where the lover's bed is perfumed with myrrh, aloe and cinnamon. It is also alluded to by Herodotus and other classical writers.

It was cinnamon that brought Dutch traders to Sri Lanka, where they established a trading post in 1638. "The shores of the island are full of it", a Dutch captain reported, "and it is the best in all the Orient: when one is downwind of the island, one can still smell cinnamon eight leagues out to sea" (Braudel 1984, p. 215).

Being a much more costly spice than cassia, that comparatively harsh-flavoured substance is frequently substituted for or added to cinnamon. The two barks when whole are easily enough distinguished, and their microscopic characteristics are also quite distinct. When powdered bark is treated with tincture of iodine (a test for starch), little effect is visible in the case of pure cinnamon of good quality, but when cassia is present a deep-blue tint is produced, the intensity of the coloration depending on the proportion of the cassia.

Culpepper's Herbal advises a daily draught of cinnamon in "any convenient liquor" against scurvy. Studies have found that using half a teaspoon of cinammon a day significantly reduces blood sugar levels in diabetics. The effect, which can even be produced by soaking cinnamon in tea, also benefits non-diabetics who have blood sugar problems.

Clinical Hold

The temporary cessation of a clinical trial by FDA if the agency is concerned about a drug or study protocol. The trial may resume when the problem is solved.

Clinical Trials

Testing of INDs (Investigational New Drugs) in human subjects to prove safety and efficacy prior to the drug's approval for marketing. The investigation of a previously untested drug is generally divided into three phases:

1. Phase I: Introducing the product (or drug) into a small number, generally 20 to 80, patients or healthy volunteers to determine the drug's metabolism, pharmacological actions, and side effects associated with increasing doses.
2. Phase II: introducing the product (or drug) into a small number, generally no more than several hundred, patients with the disease or condition under study to evaluate the effectiveness of the drug, common short-term side effects and risks associated with its use.
3. Phase III: Introducing the product (or drug) into several hundred to several thousand subjects. Studies are expanded controlled and uncontrolled trials performed after preliminary evidence suggesting effectiveness of the drug has been obtained. If the results of the Phase III Clinical Trials are

favorable, then the FDA will normally license the drug for manufacture and sale. This phase is usually performed using double blind studies with a placebo and the actual drug.
4. Phase IV: Ongoing testing studies conducted after the drug is approved. This is done to ensure the long-term efficacy of the drug, detect any long-term beneficial and/or detrimental side effects, and to determine additional potential uses for the drug.

Clone

A population of genetically identical cells derived from the multiplication of a single cell. It is the basis of rDNA and monoclonal antibody production.

Clone

A group of individuals produced from one individual through asexual processes that do not involve the interchange or combination of genetic material. As a result, members of a clone have identical genetic compositions. Protozoa and bacteria, for example, frequently reproduce asexually by a process called binary fission. In binary fission, a single-celled organism undergoes cell division and the result is two cells with identical genetic composition. Next, these two identical cells undergo division and the result is four cells with identical genetic composition. These identical offspring are all members of a clone.

Cloning

Using specialized DNA technology (also see: Cloning Vector) to produce multiple, exact copies of a single gene or other segment of DNA to obtain enough material for further study. This process is used by researchers in the Human Genome Project, and is referred to as cloning DNA. The resulting cloned (copied) collections of DNA molecules are called clone libraries. A second type of cloning exploits the natural process of cell division to make many copies of an entire cell. The genetic makeup of these cloned cells, called a cell line, is identical to the original cell. A third type of cloning produces complete, genetically identical animals such as the famous Scottish sheep, Dolly.

Cloning Vector

DNA molecule originating from a virus, a plasmid, or the cell of a higher organism into which another DNA fragment of appropriate size can be integrated without loss of the vectors capacity for self-replication; vectors introduce foreign DNA into host cells, where it can be reproduced in large quantities. Examples are plasmids, cosmids, and yeast artificial chromosomes; vectors are often recombinant molecules containing DNA sequences from several sources.

Closed System

One in which by its design and proper operation, prevents release of a microbiological agent or eukaryotic cell contained therein.

Closed System

System sterilized-in-place or sterilized while closed prior to use, is pressure or vacuum tight to some predefined leak rate, can be utilized for its intended purpose without breach to the integrity of the system, can be adapted for fluid transfers in or out while maintaining asepsis, and is connectable to other closed systems while maintaining integrity of all closed systems. (From PDA TR-28 for sterile product manufacture)

Clostridium

A genus of bacteria, most are obligate anaerobes and form endospores.

Clove

Cloves are the aromatic dried buds of a tree (Eugenia caryophyllata also sometimes Syzygium aromaticum, Myrtaceae) native to Indonesia, used as a spice in virtually all the world's cuisine. The name derives from French clou, a nail, as the buds vaguely resemble small irregular nails in shape. Cloves are harvested primarily in Indonesia and Madagascar. It is also grown in Zanzibar, India, Sri Lanka, and the "Spice Islands" (Moluccas, Indonesia known as the Bandas Islands)

Cloves can be used in cooking either whole or in a ground form, but they are extremely strong so they are used sparingly.

The spice is used throughout Europe and Asia and is smoked in cigarettes (also known as kreteks) in Indonesia and in occasional coffee bars in the West, mixed with marijuana to create marijuana spliffs, and by members of the goth subculture.

In the 3rd century BC, Chinese leaders in the Han Dynasty required those who addressed them to chew cloves so as to freshen their breath. Cloves, along with nutmeg and pepper, were highly prized to Roman times, and Pliny the Elder complained that "there is no year in which India does not drain the Roman Empire of fifty million sesterces." Cloves were traded by Arabs during the Middle Ages in the profitable Indian Ocean trade. In the late 15th century, Portugal took over the Indian Ocean trade, including cloves, due to the Treaty of Tordesillas with Spain and a separate treaty with the sultan of Ternate.

The trade later became dominated by the Dutch in the 17th century. With great difficulty the French succeeded in introducing the clove tree into Mauritius in the year 1770; subsequently the cultivation was introduced into Guiana, Brazil, most of the West Indies, and Zanzibar, where the majority of cloves today are grown.

Essential oil of clove has anesthetic and antimicrobial qualities, and is sometimes used to eliminate bad breath or to ameliorate the pain of a bad tooth. It, or its main component eugenol, is used by dentists to anesthetize the gum before injecting Novocaine or similar anesthetics, and is the characteristic odor of a dentist's office.

The clove tree is an evergreen which grows to a height ranging from 30 to 40 ft., having large oval leaves and crimson flowers in numerous groups of terminal clusters. The flower-buds are at first of a pale color and gradually become green, after which they develop into a bright red, when they are ready for collecting. Cloves are rather more than half an inch in length, and consist of a long cylindricatcalyx, terminating in four spreading sepals, and four unopened petals which form a small ball in the centre.

Antiseptic; reduces vomitting.

Coagulation

Adding insoluble compounds to water to neutralize the

electrical charge on colloids, causing them to coalesce to form larger particles that can be removed by settling.

Coaguligand

A VTA (Vascular Targeting Agent) that utilizes a human coagulation protein to induce tumor blood vessel clotting.

Coccus

A bacterium of round, spheroidal, or ovoid form, including micrococcus, staphylococcus, streptococcus, and pneumococcus.

COD (Chemical Oxygen Demand)

The amount of oxygen needed to completely oxidize all oxidizable organic and inorganic substances in water.

Coding Sequence

The region of a gene (DNA) that encodes the amino acid sequence of a protein.

Coenzyme

A non-polypeptide molecule required for the action of certain enzymes; often contains a vitamin as a component.

Cofactor

Small molecular weight, heat stable inorganic or organic substance required for the action of an enzyme.

Coliform Bacteria

A group of bacteria found in mammalian intestines and soil, used as a measure of fecal pollution in water. They are easy to identify and count in the laboratory because of their ability to ferment lactose.

Colonoscopy

Examination of the colon through a flexible, lighted instrument called a colonoscope.

Colony

A growth of microorganisms on a solid medium. The growth is visible without magnification.

Collagen

An albuminoid present in connective tissue, bone (ossein), and cartilage (chondrin), notable for its high content of the imino acids proline and hydroproxilone. On boiling with water it is converted into gelatin.

Collateral Targeting

The therapeutic strategy of targeting structures and cell types other than cancer cells common to all solid tumors as a means to attack a solid tumor.

Colloid

A translucent, yellowish material of the consistency of glue, less fluid than mucoid or mucinoid, found in the cells and tissues in a state of colloid degeneration or colloid carcinoma. A substance, such as gelatin or cytoplasm that because of the size of its molecules, is slowly diffusible rather than soluble in water and is incapable of passing through an animal membrane.

Colloids

Particles so fine they will not settle without prior coagulation. They range from 10 Å to 1,000 Å (Angstroms). They have a net negative charge and readily clog membranes and foul resin beds. Examples are bacteria, silica, and clay.

Coltsfoot (Tussilago farfara)

Soothes coughs and colds; expectorant; stimulates the immune system.

Comfrey Leaf powder (Symphytum officinale)

Impressive in speeding wound healing and guarding against scar tissue; soothes irritated surfaces; helps hemorrhages wherever they occur, internally or on the skin.

CMC (Chemistry, Manufacturing, and Controls)

The section on a BLA (Biologics License Application) or IND (Investigational New Drug) describing the composition, manufacture, and specifications of a drug product and its ingredients.

Combustible Dust

Any finely divided solid material that is 420µ or 0.017 inches or less in diameter, or any material capable of passing through an US No. 40 standard sieve that when dispersed in air in the proper proportions, could be ignited by a flame, spark or other source of ignition.

Combustible Liquid

A liquid having a closed cup flash point at or above 100°F (37.8°C). Combustible liquids do not include compressed gases or cryogenic fluids. Combustible liquids are subdivided as follows:

1. Class II - Liquids having a closed cup flash point at or above 100°F (37.8°C) and below 140°F (60°C)
2. Class III-A - liquids having a closed cup flash point at or above 140°F (60°C) and below 200°F (93.3°C)

Class III-B - liquids having a closed cup flash point at or above 200°F (93.3°C).

Commissioning

A prescribed number of activities designed to take equipment and systems from static, substantially complete state to an operable state.

Commissioning

The documented process, verifying that equipment and systems are installed according to specifications, placing the equipment and systems into active service and verifying its proper operation. Commissioning is done for good business, but can include many Qualification activities.

Complementary DNA (cDNA)

DNA that is synthesized from a messenger RNA template; the single-stranded form is often used as a probe in physical mapping.

Complementary Sequence

Nucleic acid base sequence that can form a doublestranded structure by matching base pairs with another sequence; the complementary sequence to GTAC is CATG.

Compounding

The bringing together of excipient and solvent components into a homogeneous mix of active ingredients.

Compressed Gas

A material, or mixture of materials that are either liquefied, nonliquefied, or in solution having a boiling point of 68°F (20°C) or less at 14.7 psia (101.3 kPa) of pressure. The exceptions to this rule are those gases that have no health or physical hazard properties. These gases are not considered compressed until the pressure in their packaging exceeds 41 psia (282.5 kPa) at 68°F (20°C).

Computer Controlled System

Computer system plus its controlled function.

Computer Related System

Computerized system plus its operating environment.

Computer System

A group of hardware components and associated software designed and assembled to perform a specific function or group of functions.

Computerized System

A process or operation integrated with a computer system.

Concavity (welding)

A condition in which the surface of a welded joint is depressed relative to the surface of the tube or pipe. Concavity is measured as a maximum distance from the outside or the inside diameter surface of a welded joint along a line perpendicular to a line joining the weld toes.

Concentration Polarization

The phenomenon in ultrafiltration (UF) in which solutes form a dense, polarized layer next to the membrane surface eventually blocking further flow. UF systems counteract this by continuously flushing the solute away from the membrane surface.

Concurrent Process Validation

Establishing documented evidence that a process does what it purports to do based on information generated during actual implementation of the process.

Condensate

Distillate just after it has been cooled from steam into the liquid state.

Condenser

The heat exchanger used in distillation to cool steam in order to convert it from the vapor to the liquid state.

Conductivity

The reciprocal of resistivity (C=1/R). A measure of the ability to conduct an electric current. Since ionized impurities increase the conductivity of water, it is also an accurate measure of ionic purity. Conductivity is normally expressed in micromhos/cm (µmho/cm) or microsiemens/cm (µS/cm). To measure it, current is passed between two electrodes a fixed distance apart.

Configurable Software

Commercial, off-the-shelf software that can be configured to specific user applications without altering the basic program.

Configuration

The three-dimensional shape or form of a macromolecule.

Conformation

The characteristic three-dimensional shape (tertiary structure) of a macromolecule.

Conjugated Protein

A protein containing a metal or an organic prosthetic group or both. Hemoglobin is a conjugated protein.

Consent Decree

The result of a serious violation of federal regulations and related safety and quality standards. A company must agree to a series of measures aimed at bringing its manufacturing standards in compliance with federal regulations. Until agreed-upon conditions are met, a company may be forbidden to distribute its products in interstate commerce, except for those products deemed essential for the public health.

Conserved Sequence

A base sequence in a DNA molecule (or an amino acid sequence in a protein) that has remained essentially unchanged throughout evolution.

Containment

The action of confining within a defined space a microbiological agent or other entity that is being cultured, stored, manipulated, transported, or destroyed in order to prevent or limit its contact with people and/or the environment. Methods to achieve containment include physical and biological barriers and inactivation using physical or chemical means.

1. Primary Containment. Addresses the protection of personnel and the immediate laboratory environment from exposure to infectious agents. It involves the use of closed containers or safety biological cabinets along with secure operating procedures.

2. Secondary Containment. A system of containment that prevents the escape of infectious agents into the environment external to the laboratory. It involves the use of rooms with specially designed air handling, the existence of airlocks and/or sterilizers for the exit of materials and secure operating procedures. In many cases it may add to the effectiveness of primary containment.

1. Appendix G - Physical Containment specifies physical containment for standard laboratory experiments and defines

Biosafety Level 1 (BL1) through Biosafety Level 4 (BL4). (also see: Biosafety Level, and Table II - Section II - Comparison of Good Large Scale Practice (GLSP) and Biosafety Level (BL) - Large Scale (LS) Practice)

2. Appendix I - Biological Containment specifies levels of biological containment (host vector systems) for prokaryotes and defines Host Vector 1 Systems (HV1) and Host Vector 2 Systems (HV2). (also see: Host Vector (HV) System)

3. Appendix K - Physical Containment for Large Scale Uses of Organisms Containing Recombinant DNA Molecules specifies physical containment guidelines for large scale (over 10 liters) research or production involving viable organisms containing recombinant DNA molecules, and defines GLSP (Good Large Scale Practice) through Biosafety Level 3-LS (Large Scale). (also see: Biosafety Level, and Table II - Section II - Comparison of Good Large Scale Practice (GLSP) and Biosafety Level (BL) - Large Scale (LS) Practice)

4. Appendix P - Physical and Biological Containment for Recombinant DNA Research Involving Plants specifies physical and biological containment conditions and practices suitable to the greenhouse conduct of experiments involving recombinant DNA-containing plants, plant-associated microorganisms, and small animals, and defines Biosafety Level 1-Plants (BL1-P) through Biosafety Level 4-Plants (BL4-P).

5. Appendix Q - Physical and Biological Containment for Recombinant DNA Research Involving Animals specifies containment and confinement practices for research involving whole animals, both those in which the animal's genome has been altered by stable introduction of recombinant DNA, and experiments involving viable recombinant DNA-modified microorganisms tested on whole animals, and defines Biosafety Level 1-Animals (BL1-N) through Biosafety Level 4-Animals (BL4-N).

Contaminant

Any unwanted or undesired component in a process fluid or controlled environment.

Contamination

The undesired introduction of impurities of a chemical or microbiological nature, or of foreign matter, into or onto a raw material, intermediate, or API (Active Pharmaceutical Ingredient) during production, sampling, packaging or repackaging, storage or transport.

Contig

Group of cloned (copied) pieces of DNA representing overlapping regions of a particular chromosome.

Contig Map

A map depicting the relative order of a linked library of small overlapping clones representing a complete chromosomal segment.

Continuous Fermentation

A process in which sterile medium is added without interruption to the fermentation system with a balancing withdrawal (or "harvesting") of broth for product extraction. The length of fermentation can be measured in weeks or months. Commercial applications of continuous fermentation are limited in number, with ethanol production by yeast the most important example.

Contract Manufacturer

A company holding an agreement requiring the performance of some aspect of API manufacturing

Control Area

A building or portion of a building within which the exempted amounts of hazardous materials may be stored, dispensed, handled, or used.

Control Group

The group of subjects in a controlled study that receives no treatment, receives a standard treatment, or receives a placebo.

Control Parameters

Those operating variables that can be assigned values and are used as control levels.

Control Serum

Serum used as a standard for clinical chemistry lab tests. Most often produced from outdated whole blood plasma. Most often turbid and difficult to filter

Controlled Area

An area constructed and operated in such a manner that some attempt is made to control the introduction of potential contamination, and the consequences of accidental release of living organisms. The level of control exercised should reflect the nature of the organism employed in the process. At a minimum, the area should be maintained at a pressure negative to the immediate external environment and allow for the efficient removal of small quantities of airborne contaminants.

Controlled Area

Area of restricted access. A term for areas and rooms adjoining a critical area in aseptic production facilities.

Conventional Drugs

New compounds made up by chemical synthesis or fermentation. These are termed by the FDA as NCEs (New Chemical Entities). The FDA rates conventional drugs with important therapeutic gain as 1-A drugs, for priority review. For example, AIDS drugs are conventional drugs approved for AIDS or AIDS-associated conditions.

Conventional Flow Cleanroom

A room supplied with filtered air with no specified requirement for uniform airflow patterns or velocity. Airflow patterns are usually turbulent.

Converted Data

Any original data that has been entered into a user-developed application (spreadsheet, database, report, etc.) for manipulation, evaluation, or review.

Convexity

A condition in which the surface of a welded joint is extended relative to the surface of the tube or pipe. Convexity is measured as a maximum distance from the outside or inside diameter surface of a welded joint along a line perpendicular to a line joining the weld toes.

Coriander

Coriander (Coriandrum sativum) is an annual herb commonly used in Middle Eastern, Mediterranean, Indian, Latin American, Chinese and Southeast Asian cooking. All parts of the plant are edible, but the fresh leaves and the dried seeds are the most commonly used in cooking. Coriander belongs to the parsley or carrot family, Apiaceae.

The leaves are variously referred to as **coriander leaves, cilantro** (in the United States, from the Spanish name for the plant), **dhania** (in the Indian subcontinent, and increasingly, in Britain), **Chinese parsley** or **Mexican parsley**. The leaves have a very different taste from the seeds. Some people consider the taste offensive and describe it as soapy. The difference in perception of the flavor of the leaves may have a genetic cause and is so common that a website has been established based on the phenomenon.

The fresh leaves are an essential ingredient in many Asian chutneys and Mexican salsas and guacamole. Chopped coriander leaves are also used as a garnish on cooked dishes such as dal and many curries, but should never themselves be cooked as heat destroys their delicate flavor quickly.

The fresh herb is best stored in the refrigerator in air tight containers, after chopping off the roots.

The seeds are known as coriander seeds and have a lemon citrus flavor when crushed. It is also described as warm, nutty, spicy, and orange-flavoured. They are usually dried but can be eaten green. Ground coriander is a major ingredient in curry powder, certain belgian style beers and other aromatic dishes.

If the spice is bought whole in a non-dried form, it can be dried in the sun. Most commonly, it is bought as whole dried seeds, but can be bought in ground form. Store coriander seed in a tightly sealed container away from sunlight and heat. For maximum flavor use within 6 months and keep for no more than 1 year. It can be roasted or heated on a dry pan briefly to enhance the aroma before grinding it in an electric grinder or with a mortar and pestle; ground coriander seeds lose their flavour quickly in storage and are best only ground as needed. It is a key ingredient in Indian curries and garam masala (Hindi name: *dhania).* It is also used in Ethiopian and Arabic cooking.

It is believed to have originated in the Mediterranean area, and in Southwest Europe. Some believe its use began as far back as 5,000 BC, and there is evidence of its use by the Egyptians. In the Bible, Exodus, chapter 16, verse 31, it says that: "And the house of Israel called the name there of Manna: and it was like coriander seed, white; and the taste of it was like wafers made with honey". Coriander was brought to the United States of America in 1670 and was one of the first spices cultivated by early settlers.

Coriander seed and leaf was very widely used in medieval European cuisine, due to its ability to make spoiled meats palatable by "masking" rotten flavors. Even today, coriander seed is an important ingredient in many sausage products.

The name coriander, coriandrum, first noted by Pliny, derives from Greek Corys (a bedbug), + -ander (resembling), and refers to the supposed similarity of the scent of the crushed leaves to the distinctive odor of bedbugs (which we have largely forgotten in this age of insecticides).

Corn Steep Liquor

An ingredient in the culture medium for producing penicillin. A natural nitrogenous material that is a by-product of the corn milling industry.

Corrosive

A chemical that causes visible destruction or irreversible alterations in living tissue by chemical action at the site of contact. A chemical is considered corrosive if, when tested on the intact skin of albino rabbits by the method described in Appendix A of CFR 49 Part 173, it destroys or changes irreversibly the structure of the tissue at the site of contact following an exposure period of four hours. This term shall not refer to action on inanimate surfaces.

Corrosive Liquid

A liquid which when in contact with living tissue, will cause destruction or irreversible alteration of such tissue by chemical action. Examples include acidic, alkaline, or caustic materials.

Cosmid

Artificially constructed cloning vector containing the cos gene of phage lambda. Cosmids can be packaged in lambda p0hage particles for infection into E. coli: this permits cloning of larger DNA fragments (up to 45kb) that can be introduced into bacterial hosts in plasmid vectors.

CP (Cyclic Polarization)

An electrochemical test (ASTM G61) for metals that measures the point at which pitting corrosion begins. CP uses an electrolytic cell to directly measure the corrosion rate. By using the test piece as the working electrode, initiation of localized corrosion is shown by the potential at which the current density increases rapidly. This point is called the "pitting potential". The lower the current density at this point, the more resistance to pitting corrosion. The current density is measured in micro-amps per square centimeter.

Cramp Bark (Viburnum opulus)

Relaxes muscle tensions and reduces spasms; relaxes the uterus and relieve painful menstrual cramps; helps to prevent menstrual excessive blood loss; protects from threatened miscarriage; sedative.

Critical

A material, process step, or process condition, test requirement, or any other relevant parameter is considered critical when non-compliance with predetermined criteria directly influences the quality attributes of the API (Active Pharmaceutical Ingredient) in a detrimental manner.

Critical Area

An area where (sterile) product or contact surface is exposed, normally Class 100 (e.g., Point of Fill).

Critical Device

A device that directly ensures that a GMP Critical Parameter is maintained within predetermined limits (e.g., terminal HEPA filter, point of use filter). A malfunction of such a device would place product quality directly at risk.

Critical Instrument

An instrument that measures a GMP Critical Parameter, used to monitor and document that parameter.

Critical Parameter

A GMP or product quality parameter (e.g., differential pressure, unidirectional airflow pattern) that must be maintained within predefined limits to ensure product SISPQ (Strength, Identity, Safety, Purity, or Quality).

Critical Point

The combination of pressure and temperature at which the gas and liquid phases of a substance become indistinguishable.

Critical Process Step

For sterile products, this normally is an activity where product or product contact parts are exposed to the surrounding environment.

Critical Step(s)

The point or points in the process which, if not carried out properly or if contaminated, will not allow drug substances to be made such that they will meet their intended characterizations and impurity profiles.

Critical Surface

The part of the working surface to be protected from particulate contamination. It is within the Critical Zone.

Critical System

A structural, mechanical, or electrical system that can impact the processing parameters and attributes of the finished product or regulatory study. Critical systems may include utilities, process equipment, and systems.

Cross Contamination

The measurable and detrimental contamination of a material or product with another material or product.

Crossing Over

The breaking during meiosis of one maternal and one paternal chromosome, the exchanging of corresponding sections of DNA, and the rejoining of the chromosomes. This process can result in an exchange of alleles between chromosomes.

Cryogenic Liquid

A fluid that has a normal boiling point below -150°F (-101.1°C).

Cryptography

The mathematical science of deliberately scrambling and unscrambling information. Information is protected by being transformed (encrypted) into an unreadable format, called cipher text. Only those who posses a secret key can decypher (or decrypt) that message into plain text.

Culture Medium

Any nutrient system for the artificial cultivation of bacteria or other cells; usually a complex mixture of organic and inorganic materials.

Cumin

Cumin (Cuminum cyminum) is a plant and a spice with a distinctive aroma, popular in Mexican, North African, and Indian cuisine. It belongs to the family Apiaceae, which is popularly called the carrot family.

Cumin has been grown and used as a spice since ancient times. Originally cultivated in Iran and the Mediterranean region, cumin is mentioned in the Bible in both the Old Testament (Isaiah 28:27) and in the New Testament (Matthew 23:23). It was also known in ancient Greece and Rome. The Greeks kept cumin at the dining table in its own container -

much as pepper is frequently kept today - and this practice continues in Morocco. Cumin fell out of favor in Europe (except in Spain) during the Middle Ages, but is widely used today. It is now mostly grown in Morocco, Egypt, India, Syria, North America, and Chile.

The name cumin is a distortion of the Persian city Kerman, where most of ancient Persia's cumin was produced. For the Persians the expression carrying "cumin to Kerman" means: "to carry coal to Newcastle". Kerman, locally called Kermun, became Kumun and then cumin in the European languages. In India, cumin is known as jeera.

The cumin plant is an annual herb. Its stem is slender and branching to about a foot in height; the leaves are laciniate with filiform segments; the flowers are small, white or pink, and borne in umbels. The so-called seeds are its fruits, which are achenes. These, which constitute the spice cumin, are fusiform or ovoid in shape, and compressed laterally. Cumin seeds looks similar to fennel seeds, but are smaller and darker in color.

Cumin fruits have a distinctive bitter flavor and strong, warm aroma due to their abundant essential oil content. Its main constituent and important aroma compound is cuminaldehyde (4-isopropylbenzaldehyde). Important aroma compounds of toasted cumin are the substituted pyrazines, 2-ethoxy-3-isopropylpyrazine, 2-methoxy-3-sec-butylpyrazine, and 2-methoxy-3-methylpyrazine. Their smell can also be detected in the eater's sweat even after consuming only small amounts.

Today, cumin is identified with Indian cuisine and Mexican cuisine. It is used as an ingredient of curry powder. Cumin can be found in some Dutch cheeses, and in some traditional breads from France. In herbal medicine, cumin is classified as stimulant, carminative, and antimicrobial.

Cumin is hotter to the taste, lighter in colour, and larger than caraway (Carum carvi), another umbelliferous spice that is sometimes confused with it. Cumin is also not related to black cumin, which is an alternate name for nigella (Nigella sativa).

Curry Tree

The Curry Tree, Curry-leaf Tree, or Curry Patta (Murraya koenigii; sometimes classified as Bergera koenigii or Chalcas

koenigii), is a species in the family Rutaceae.
This tropical to sub-tropical tree is native to India, where its leaves are used as a herb. The tree grows 2-5 m tall, with small white, fragrant flowers. The small black, shiny berries are claimed to be edible, but their seeds are claimed to be poisonous. The leaves of the curry tree must be used fresh, as they lose their flavour when dried.

Cut

An enzymatic break that occurs in both strands of a DNA molecule opposite one another by restriction enzymes.

Cystic Fibrosis

An inherited disease in which thick mucus clogs the lungs and blocks the ducts of the pancreas.

Cytokine

A protein that acts as a chemical messenger to stimulate cell migration, usually toward where the protein is released. Interlukins, lymphokines, and interferons are the most common.
2. Group of extracellular factors produced by a variety of cells including monocytes, lymphocytes, and non-lymphoid cells. Cytokines include the interleukins, some interferons, and tumor necrosis factor. They are important in controlling local and systemic inflammatory response.

Cytolysis

The dissolution of cells particularly by destruction of their cell membrane.

Cytopathic

Damaging to cells.

Cytoplasm

The protoplasmic contents of the cell outside the nucleus in which the cell's organelles are suspended.

Cytosine (C)
A pyrimidine occurring as a fundamental unit or base of nucleic acids.

Cytostatic Agents
Therapeutics that inhibit cell division and growth. This term can refer to machinery, such as those that would freeze cells.

Cytotoxic
Poisonous to cells.

Cytotoxicity
The ability of a substance or compound to cause a cytotoxic effect.

D

Dandelion (Taraxacum officinale)
Treats liver infections and breast cancer36; helpful in detoxifying the liver.

Dalton
The unit of molecular weight, equal to the weight of a hydrogen atom.

Data Integrity
The validity of data and their relationships. For electronic records to be trustworthy and reliable, the links between raw data, metadata, and results must not be compromised or broken. Without data integrity, it is not possible to regenerate a previous result reliably.

Data Migration
The process of translating data from one system to another when a company replaces the current computing systems with a new one. CFR 21 Part 11 mandates that data migration implementation create accurate and complete copies of the records when they are moved to a new system.

DDC (Direct Digital Control)
A collection of control units (analog and discrete) connected into a data highway, usually with a host or alarming/ recording computer attached.

D Value

The time under a stated set of exposure conditions (temperature in an autoclave) required to reduce a microbial population by a factor of 90% (e.g. from 10,000 to 1,000).

Dead Leg

An area of entrapment in a vessel or piping run that could lead to contamination of the product. In a piping system, a non-flowing pocket, tee, or extension from a primary piping run that exceeds a defined number of pipe diameters from the ID of the primary pipe. Denoted by the term L/D or L/A, where L is equal to the leg extension perpendicular to the normal flow pattern or direction, A is the annular gap width, and D is equal to the ID (or inside dimension) of the extension or leg. In some existing standards, the dimension L is measured from the centerline of the primary pipe. For bioprocessing systems, an L/D of 2:1 is achievable with today's component technology for most valving and piping configurations.

Decontamination

A process that reduces contaminating substances to a defined acceptance level.

Deflagration

An exothermic reaction, such as the extremely rapid oxidation of a combustible dust or flammable vapor in air, in which the reaction progresses through the unburned material at a rate less than the velocity of sound. A deflagration can have an explosive effect.

Deglycosylation

The removal of a sugar unit (i.e., glucose) from a larger molecule called a glycoside. For example, an enzyme called beta-glycosidase removes the sugar unit from the isoflavone glycoside daidzin, leaving the aglycone, daidzein.

Degrading

Deterioration of a surface finish so that pieces of the finish (or substrate) material large enough to be visible to the unaided eye, dislodge without any direct physical contact and fall from the surface of the material.

Deionization

Removing dissolved ions from solution by passing the solution through a bed of ion exchange resin, consisting of polymer beads that exchange hydrogen ions for cations and hydroxyl ions for anions in solution. The ionic impurities remain bound to the resins and the hydrogen and hydroxyl ions combine with each other to form water.

Deletion Map

A description of a specific chromosome that uses defined mutations - specific deleted areas in the genome - as "biochemical signposts", or markers for specific areas.

De Minimis Release

The release of viable microbiological agents or eukaryotic cells that does not result in the establishment of disease in healthy people, plants, or animals; or in uncontrolled proliferation of any microbiological agents or eukaryotic cells.

Dementia

Severe impairment of mental functioning.

Demineralization

Sometimes used interchangeably with deionization, it refers to the removal of minerals and mineral salts using ion exchange. Water softening is a common form of demineralization.

Demethylation

The removal of a methyl group ($-CH_3$) from a molecule; for example, when the methyl group is removed from the isoflavone biochanin A, the resulting molecule is called genistein.

Denaturation

The loss of the native structure of a macromolecule resulting, from heat treatment, extreme pH changes, chemical treatment, etc. It is accompanied by loss of biological activity. For example, proteins may be denatured by heat, pH extremes, or addition of agents such as urea or guanidinium hydrochloride.

Dent

A typical stainless steel interior surface anomaly that refers to a large, smooth-bottomed depression whose diameter or width is greater than its depth and which will not produce an indication.

Depyrogenation

The removal or destruction of endotoxins.

Derivative

Chemicals which are made from their parent compounds are known as derivatives of the parent compound.

Desalination

The removal of dissolved salts from brine to produce potable water.

Design Condition

The specified range or accuracy of a controlled variable used by the designer to determine performance requirements of an engineered system.

Design Specification

A specification that defines the design of a system or system component.

Desiccant

Chemical salt used to dehumidify air, to control moisture in materials contacting that air.

Desiccators

Closed containers, usually made of glass or plastic, with an airtight seal used for drying materials.

Detonation

An exothermic reaction characterized by the presence of a shock wave in a material that establishes and maintains the reaction. The reaction zone progresses through the material at a rate greater than the velocity of sound. The principal heating mechanism is one of shock compression. Detonations have an explosive effect.

Deuteromycetes

Molds that cannot reproduce by sexual means. Some pathogenic fungi such as Trichophyton, which causes athlete's foot, belong to this family.

DHL Vaccine

A tri-valent vaccine. Also, the most common veterinary vaccine that has a combination of viral and bacterial vaccines. Used for distemper, hepatitis (canine), and leptospira.

Diagnostic

A substance or group of substances used to identify a disease by analyzing the cause and symptoms.

Dialysis

The separation of low-molecular weight compounds from high molecular weight components by diffusion through a semipermeable membrane. Frequently utilized to remove salts, introduce salts, remove biological effectors such as nicotinamide adenine dinucleotides, nucleotides phosphates, etc. from polymeric molecules such as protein, DNA, RNA, etc. Commonly used membranes have a molecular weight cutoff around 10,000 but other membrane pore sizes are available.

Diatom

Any minute, unicellular or colonial algae of the class Bacillariophyceae having siliceous cells walls consisting of two overlapping symmetrical parts.

Diffusion

The random thermal motion of particles, which causes them to flow from a region of higher concentration to one of lower concentration until they are uniformly distributed.

Digestion

The enzymatic hydrolysis of major nutrients in the

gastrointestinal system to yield their building-block components.

Digitalis

A series of on and off pulses arranged to convey information.

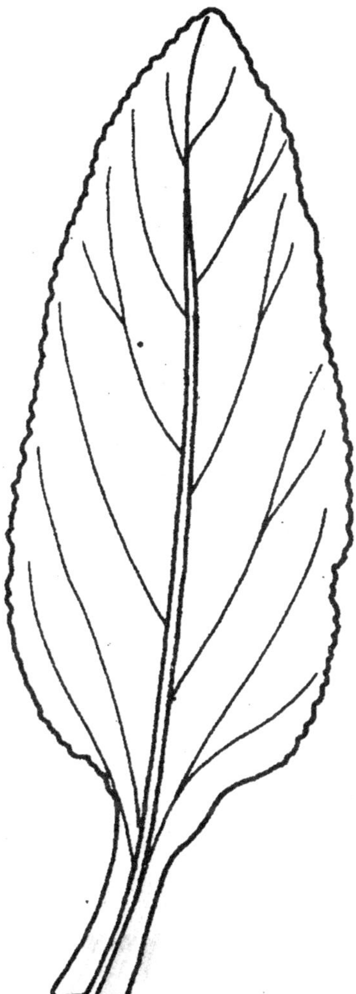

Digitalis Leaf

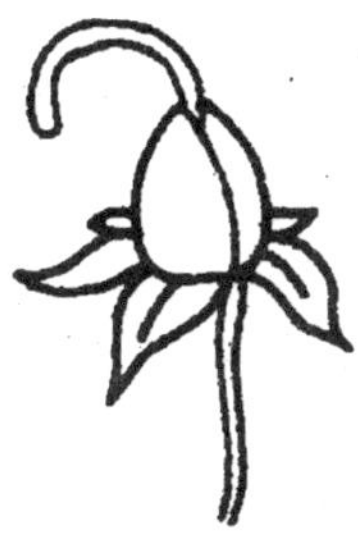

Fruit

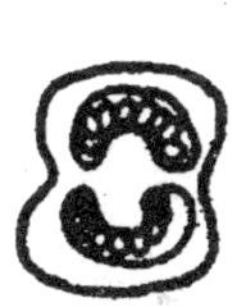

Ovary

Digital Certificate

An attachment to an electronic message used for security purposes. The most common use of a digital certificate is to verify that a user sending a message is who he or she claims to be and to provide the receiver with the means to encode a reply.

Digital Representation

Biometric parameters such as a fingerprint or retinal pattern are turned into data that a computer understands: the digital representation of the biometric. The pattern in the biometric divides it into a grid of boxes, and a zero or a one, depending on whether the box is filled in, marks each box.

Digital Signature

An electronic signature based upon cryptographic methods of originator authentication, computed by using a set of rules and a set of parameters such that the identity of the signer and the integrity of the data can be verified.

Dill

Dill (Anethum graveolens) is a short-lived, European, annual herb. Dill seeds are used to flavor pickles; the fernlike leaves (called dill weed) are used to flavor many other foods, such as borscht. It is an umbelliferous plant, very like the caraway, its leaves, which are aromatic, being used in soups and pickles. This name dill is derived from a Norse word which means to soothe, the plant having the carminative property of allaying pain. The common dill, Anethum graveolens, is an annual growing wild in the cornfields of Spain and Portugal and the south of Europe generally.

There is also a species of dill cultivated in Eastern countries known by the name of shubit. It was this species of garden plant of which the Pharisees were in the habit of paying tithes. The Talmud requires that the seeds, leaves, and stem of dill shall pay tithes. Jesus rebuked them for tithing dill but omitting mercy.

Classification: Dill is a member of the parsley or carrot family, Apiaceae (formerly Umbelliferae).

Dill can grow it at least USDA Plant Hardiness Zones 7.

While it prefers sun, even in partial shaded areas a crop of seeds can be harvested.
Helps eliminate gas in infants; tranquilizer; softens hardened stools.

Dilution

Lowering the concentration of a solution by adding more solvent.

Dilution Factor

The ratio of solvent to solute by volume.

Diploid

A full set of genetic material, consisting of paired chromosomes one chromosome from each parental set. Most animal cells except the gametes have a diploid set of chromosomes. The diploid human genome has 46 chromosomes.

Diplophase

A phase in the life cycle of an organism where the organism has two copies of each gene. The organism is said to be diploid.

Direct Impact System

An engineering system that may have a direct impact on product quality.

Disaster

Any event (i.e. fire, earthquake, power failure etc.), which could have a detrimental effect upon an automated system or its associated information.

Discoloration (welding)

Any change in surface color from that of the base metal. Usually associated with oxidation occurring on the weld and heat affected zone (HAZ) on the outside diameter and inside diameter of the weld joint as a result of heating the metal during the welding. Colors may range from pale bluish-gray to deep blue, and from pale straw color to a black crusty coating.

Disinfection

Process by which viable microbiological agents or eukaryotic cells are reduced to a level unlikely to produce disease in healthy people, plants, or animals. These processes may use chemical agents, heat, ultraviolet light, etc. to destroy most (but not necessarily all) of the harmful or objectionable microorganisms, pathogens, and potential pathogens. Disinfection does not necessarily result in sterilization.

1. "High level disinfection" inactivates fungi, viruses, and bacteria. High-level chemical disinfectants maybe ineffective against bacterial spores if they are present in large numbers. Extended exposure times may be required.
2. "Intermediate level disinfection" destroys fungi, some viruses (lipid and most non-lipid medium-size and small viruses), mycobacteria, and bacteria.
3. "Low level disinfection" kills vegetative forms of bacteria, some fungi, and some medium-size and lipid-containing viruses. Low-level disinfectants do not reliably kill bacterial spores, mycobacteria, or small or non-lipid viruses.

Dispensing

The pouring or transferring of any material from a container, tank or similar vessel, whereby vapors, dusts, fumes, mists or gases may be liberated to the atmosphere.

Dissimilation

The breakdown of food material to yield energy and building blocks for cellular synthesis.

Dissolved Solids

The amount of nonvolatile matter dissolved in a water sample, usually expressed in parts per million (PPM) by weight.

Distillation

The process of separating water from impurities by heating until it changes into vapor and then cooling the vapor to condense it into purified water.

DNA (Deoxyribonucleic Acid)

The molecule of which the genetic material is composed. It

consists of two chains joined together as a double helix. Each chain is composed of a polymer of nucleotides (consisting of a nitrogenous base, a deoxyribosesugar ring, and a phosphate group) joined together by phosphodiester bonds between the 5'-phosphate of one nucleotide and the 3'-hydroxyl of the next. The two chains run in opposite directions and are held together by hydrogen bonds between the bases in equivalent positions in the two chains. There are various forms of double helical DNA. They are:

1. B-DNA (first described by Crick and Watson) is a right-handed helix with 10.6 base pairs per turn and is probably the main form of cellular DNA.
2. A-DNA is also a right-handed helix but is somewhat skewed and contains about 11 base pairs per turn. It is the form taken By DNA-RNA hybrid double helixes.
3. Z-DNA is a left-handed helix with 11 base pairs per turn. It is favored by regions rich in guanine cutosine base pairs and probably occurs infrequently in cellular DNA.

DNA (Deoxyribonucleic Acid)

The molecular basis for genes; every inherited characteristic has its origin somewhere in the code of the organism's complement of DNA. The code is made up of subunits, nucleic acids. The organism to produce the required proteins that compose the genetic traits of the organism and its life functions interprets the sequence of the four nucleic acids.

DNAse (Deoxyribonuclease)

An enzyme that degrades DNA.

DNA Array

Spots of DNA arranged on a slide support such as glass or silicon "DNA chip" (or microarray), used for screening, sequencing, genetic mapping, and so on.

DNA Replication

The use of existing DNA as a template for the synthesis of new DNA strands. In humans and other eukaryotes, replication occurs in the cell nucleus.

DNA Sequence

The relative order of base pairs, whether in a fragment of DNA, a gene, a chromosome, or an entire genome. (also see:

DNA Vector

A DNA vehicle for transferring generic information from one cell to another.

Documentation Written or pictorial information describing, defining, specifying, and/or reporting of certifying activities, requirements, procedures or results.

Domain

A discrete portion of a protein with its own function. The combination of domains in a single protein determines its overall function.

Dominant Allele

A gene that is expressed, regardless of whether its counterpart allele on the other chromosome is dominant or recessive. Autosomal dominant disorders are produced by a single mutated dominant allele, even though its corresponding allele is normal.

Dose Response

Change in response of organisms related to changes in overall exposure to substance.

DOP (Dioctyl Phthalate)

A mono-dispersed test aerosol of sub-micron particles, generated to challenge (evaluate integrity) of HEPA filters for HVAC.

DOP (Dispersed Oil Particulate)

(also see: DOP (Dioctyl Phthalate))

Dosage Form

The form in which the drug is delivered to the patient. This could be parenteral, topical, tablet, oral (liquid or dissolved powder), suppository, inhalation, transdermal, etc.

Dosage Group

A group of subjects in a clinical trial receiving the same dosage (amount) of a drug being tested.

Double-blind

Experimental design protocol in which neither the subject nor the investigator(s) working with the subject or analysing data know what treatment, if any, the subject is receiving. At the end of the experiment, the "code" is broken and the data analysed with respect to the various treatments.

Double Blind Test

Used in Clinical Trials, this is a method to ensure that any one party cannot improperly influence the test. The product (either in a single strength dosage or in multiple dosages) and the placebo are packaged and given a code name known to only the initiating party. These are then sent to another party who gives the coded packages yet another code name or number, and makes a matrix of the previous name/number to the new name/number. This is then sent to the physician who administers these to the patient. At the end of the test, the physician provides records of which patient received which code name/number product. This is then cross-referenced to the intermediate matrix to determine the original code name/number. The results of the treatment are then correlated to determine the efficacy of the drug.

The structure of DNA as proposed by Watson and Crick. It consists of two right-handed helical polynucleotide chains coiled around the same axis. The two chains are anti-parallel with their 3rd to 5th internucleotide phosphodiester bonds running in opposite directions. Under most conditions, the coiling of the chains is such that if the ends are held still, as in circular DNA or in a large chromosome, the chains cannot be separated except by cleavage of one of the strands.

Double bond

Atoms are sharing two pairs of electrons in a double bond. This kind of bond is therefore called 'electron rich.' A double bond can become the site of chemical reactions. For example, this sulfide molecule from Garlic has a double bond at each end, represented by the double lines. (Each angle in the drawing represents a carbon atom; there is also a carbon atom at each end of the double lines).

Drugs

Articles intended for use in diagnosis, cure, mitigation, treatment, or prevention of disease in man or other animals" and "articles (other than food) intended to affect the structure or any function of the body of man or other animals.

Drug Product

A finished dosage form, for example, tablet, capsule, solution, etc., that contains one or more APIs (Active Pharmaceutical Ingredients) generally, but not necessarily, in association with inactive ingredients. The term also includes a finished dosage form, which does not contain an API but is intended to be used as a placebo.

Drug (Medicinal) Product

The dosage form in the final immediate packaging intended for marketing.

Dry Air

Air from which all water vapor and contaminants have been removed. Its composition by volume is:

1. Nitrogen 78.08%
2. Oxygen 20.95%
3. Argon 0.93%
4. Carbon Dioxide 0.03
5. Other gases 0.00003

Dry Heat Sterilization

Sterilization utilizing a heating oven or continuous tunnel (gas or electric heated), as opposed to steam sterilization in an autoclave, usually used for glassware and metal parts. In depyrogenation temperatures of 250°C result in sterilization and the inactivation of endotoxin present on the surface of the equipment.

Durability

The ability to withstand the rigors of the environment without degrading or requiring repair.

Dust (also see: Combustible Dust)

Dusting Deterioration of the finish at the surface so it is easily loosened from the surface by light physical contact (such as wiping one's hand across the surface), mechanically induced air movements or naturally occurring air movements.

Dynamic Conditions

Environmental conditions of a manufacturing room occupied by the normal number of workers appropriately garbed and with production equipment in operation. However, dynamic conditions for some dusty operations, such as aseptic powder filling, may be measured in the absence of product.

E Coli (Escherichia Coli)

A fast growing, Gram-negative bacteria commonly found in the body with a comparatively simple structure. The genetic make up of E. coli is the best known of any organism, having been widely studied during the development of genetic engineering. It has been used extensively as the host cell for novel proteins made by rDNA technology.

E

Echinacea (Echinacea Angustifolia)

An immune stimulant and the liquid extract is sweet tasting.

Echinacea (Echinacea purperea)

An immune stimulant by increasing phagocytosis37; used to treat fevers and minor infections.

Ecological Succession

The gradual process by which species composition of an ecosystem change.

Ecology

The study of the interrelationships between organisms and their environment.

Ecosystem

The interaction of all living organisms in a particular environment.

Edge Failure

A control parameter value that, if exceeded, may result in adverse effect on state of control and/or fitness for use of the product.

Efficacy

The ability of a substance to produce a desired effect.

Effluent

The output or discharge from a process, such as a wastewater treatment process.

Elastin

An albuminoid, or scleroprotein present especially in yellow elastic fibrous tissue.

Elastomer

Long chain co-polymers or terpolymers (two or three different monomers in one chain) that contain adequate crosslinks among individual chains. Fluorinated elastomers are more stable than hydrocarbon or silicon elastomers because C-F bonds are approximately 30% stronger than C-H bonds. There are five major FDA compliant elastomers used in the pharmaceutical and biopharmaceutical industries: EPDM (ethylene-propylene-diene rubber), fluororelastomers (FKM), platinum-cured silicon (pt-Si), and finally Kalrez® parts using compounds KLR-6221 and KLR-6230, which are perfluoroelastomers.

Elastomeric Material

A material that can be stretched or compressed repeatedly and, upon immediate release of stress, will return to its approximate original size.

Elder flowers (Sambucus canadensis)

Releives symptoms of coughs and colds

Elderberry

Elder or Elderberry *(Sambucus)* is a genus of between 5-30 species of fast-growing shrubs or small trees (two species herbaceous) formerly treated in the honeysuckle family Caprifoliaceae, but now shown by genetic evidence to be correctly classified in the moschatel family (Adoxaceae).

The leaves are opposite, pinnate, with 5-9 leaflets (rarely 3 or 11), each leaf 5-30 cm long, the leaflets with a serrated margin. They bear large bunches of small white or cream coloured flowers in the late spring, that are followed by bunches of small red, bluish or black berries. The berries are a very valuable food resource for many birds and the flowers are eaten by the larva of The V-Pug moth. The crushed foliage and immature fruit have a strong foetid smell.

The **common elder** complex is variously treated as a single species *Sambucus nigra* found in the warmer parts of Europe and North America with several regional varieties or subspecies, or else as a group of several similar species. The flowers are in flat umbels, and the berries are black to glaucous blue; they are larger shrubs, reaching 5-8 m tall, occasionally small trees up to 15 m tall and with a stem diameter of up to 30-60 cm.

Applied externally for burns, rashes, and minor skin problems.

Elecampane root (Inula helenium)

Diuretic; diaphoretic; helps with coughs, and bronchitis.

Electrical Area Classifications

Facilities, or portions of facilities are classified electrically according to the type of material present and its flammability and/or explosive potential. Each area classification carries with it specific requirements for the construction requirements found within that space to guard against sparking. The Class of an area refers to the type of material; the Division of the area refers to whether that material is normally found in that area or not. Electrical classifications are covered by the National Electrical Code (NEC) adopted by the National Fire Protection Association (NFPA) as Volume 6 of the National Fire Codes. They are:

1. Class I, Division 1: A Class I, Division 1 location (1) is that in which ignitable concentrations of flammable gases/vapors can exist under normal operating conditions; or (2) in which ignitable concentrations of such gases/vapors may exist frequently because of repair, maintenance operations or because of leakage; or (3) in which breakdown or faulty operation of equipment or process may release ignitable concentrations of flammable gases/vapors, and might also cause simultaneous failure of electric equipment. 2. Class I, Division

2: A Class I, Division 2 location (1) is that in which volatile flammable liquids or flammable gases are handled, processed, or used, but in which the liquids, vapors, or gases will normally be confined within closed containers or closed systems from which they can escape only in case of accidental rupture or breakdown of such containers or systems, or in case of abnormal operation of equipment; or (2) in which ignitable concentrations of gases or vapors are normally prevented by positive mechanical ventilation, and which might become hazardous through failure or abnormal operation of the ventilating equipment; or (3) that is adjacent to a class I, Division 1 location, and to which ignitable concentrations of gases or vapors might occasionally be communicated unless such communication is prevented by adequate positive-pressure ventilation from a source of clean air, and effective safeguards against ventilation failure are provided.

3. Class II, Division 1: A Class II, Division 1 location (1) is that in which combustible dust is in the air under normal operating conditions in quantities sufficient to produce explosive or ignitable mixtures; or (2) where mechanical failure or abnormal operation of machinery or equipment might cause such explosive or ignitable mixtures to be produced, and might also provide a source of ignition through simultaneous failure of electric equipment, operation of protection device, or from other causes; or (3) in which combustible dusts of an electrically conductive nature may be present in hazardous quantities.

4. Class II, Division 2: A Class II, Division 2 location (1) is that in which combustible dust is not normally in the air in quantities sufficient to produce explosive or ignitable mixtures, and dust accumulations are normally insufficient to interfere with the normal operation of electrical equipment or other apparatus but combustible dust may be in suspension in the air as a result of infrequent malfunctioning of handling or processing equipment and where combustible dust accumulations on, in, or in the vicinity of the electrical equipment may be sufficient to interfere with the safe dissipation of heat from electrical equipment or may be ignitable by abnormal operation or failure of electrical equipment.

5. Class III, Division 1: A Class III, Division 1 location is that in which easily ignitable fibers or materials producing combustible filings are handled, manufactured, or used.

6. Class III, Division 2: Class III, Division 2 location is that in which easily ignitable fibers are stored or handled.

Electrical Code

Electrical Groups Electrical groupings are based on the characteristics of the materials involved. These include the following:

1. Class I, Group A: Atmospheres containing acetylene.
2. Class I, Group B: Atmospheres containing hydrogen, fuel and combustible process gases containing more than 30 percent hydrogen by volume, or gases or vapors of equivalent hazard such as butadiene, ethylene oxide, propylene oxide, and acrolein.
3. Class I, Group C: Atmospheres such as ethyl ether, ethylene, or gases or vapors of equivalent hazard.
4. Class I, Group D: Atmospheres such as acetone, ammonia, benzene, butane, cyclopropane, ethanol, gasoline, hexane, methanol, methane, natural gas, naphtha, propane, or gases or vapors of equivalent hazard.
5. Class II, Group E: Atmospheres containing combustible metal dusts, including aluminum, magnesium and their commercial alloys, or other combustible dusts whose particle size, abrasiveness, and conductivity present similar hazards in the use of electrical equipment.
6. Class II, Group F: Atmospheres containing combustible carbonaceous dusts, including carbon black, charcoal, coal, or coke dusts that have more that 8 percent entrapped volatiles, or dusts that have been sensitized by other materials so that they present an explosion hazard.
7. Class II, Group G: Atmospheres containing combustibles dusts not included in Group E or F, including flour, grain, wood, plastic, and chemicals.

Electrodialysis (ED)

A membrane separation method used for the separation of charged molecules from a solution by application of a direct current. The membranes contain ion-exchange groups and have a fixed electrical charge. This method is very effective in the concentration of electrolytes and proteins.

Electrolyte

A chemical compound which when dissolved or ionized in water allows it to conduct electric current.

Electron Microscopy (EM)

A technique for visualizing material that uses beams of electrons instead of light rays and that permits greater magnification than is possible with an optical microscope. Electron microscopes have been used to examine the structure of viruses and bacteria, to identify and classify pollen grains, etc.

Electronic Record

Any combination of text, graphics, data, audio, pictorial, or other information representation in digital form that is created, modified, maintained, archived, retrieved, or distributed by a computer system.

Electronic Signature or e-sig

According to FDA, an electronic signature is a computer data compilation of any symbol or series of symbols executed, adopted, or authorized by an individual to be the legally binding equivalent of the individual's handwritten signature.

Electrophoresis

The migration of electrically charged proteins, colloids, molecules, or other particles when dissolved or suspended in an electrolyte through which an electric current is passed. The most important use of electrophoresis is in the analysis of blood proteins. Since the proportion of these proteins varies widely in different diseases, electrophoresis can be used for diagnostic purposes. Electrophoresis is used to study bacteria and viruses, nucleic acids, and some types of smaller molecules, including amino acids.

Electropolishing

Also known as "chemical machining" and "reverse plating", electropolishing is an electrochemical process far superior to any available mechanical process for the removal of minute surface imperfections in stainless steel. It levels and brightens the material surface by anodic dissolution in an electrolyte flowing solution with an imposed electrical current. When the proper combination of electrolyte current & temperature is attained, the high points of surface irregularities, or high current density areas, are selectively removed at a greater rate than the remainder of the surface, resulting in improved surface smoothness. During electropolishing, the polarized surface film is subjected to the combined effects of gassing (oxygen) that occurs with electromechanical metal removal, saturation of the surface with dissolved metal, and the agitation and temperature of the electrolyte.

Electrolyte

Any compound which in solution conducts a current of electricity and is decomposed by it.

Electrostatic Fluidized Bed

A container holding powder coating material which is aerated from below so as to form an air-supported expanded cloud of such material which is electrically charged with a charge opposite to the charge of the object to be coated. Such object is transported through the container immediately above the charged and aerated materials in order to be coated.

ELISA (Enzyme Linked Immunosorbent Assay)

A test to measure the concentration of antigens or antibodies.

Elute

To separate one solute from another by washing. Elution may include the removal by means of a suitable solvent of one material (absorbed material) from another (adsorbent) that is insoluble in that solvent.

Ellinghausen's Medium

A complex medium for growing Leptospira (also see; DHL vaccine). Contains numerous salts, nutrients, and BSA (Bovine Serum Albumin).

Embriology

The study of the early stages in the development of an organism. In these stages a single highly specialized cell, the egg, is transformed into a complex, many-celled organism resembling its parents.

Endemic

A disease present in a community or among a group of people; used to describe a disease prevailing continually in a region.

Endergonic Reaction

A chemical reaction with a positive standard free energy change, an "uphill" reaction.

Endocrine Glands

The glands that secrete their products (hormones) into the blood that then carries them to their specific target organs. Endocrine glands are the pituitary, thyroids, adrenals, pancreas, ovaries (in females), and testes (in males). Endocrine glands are found in some invertebrates as well as in vertebrates.

Endocrine Hormones

The products secreted by the endocrine glands. These help control long-term processes, such as growth, lactation, sex cycles, and metabolic adjustment. The endocrine system and the nervous system are interdependent and are often referred to collectively as the neuroendocrine system. For example, the juvenile hormone, found in insects and annelids, affects sexual maturation. There is currently great interest in the possible use of such hormones in the control of destructive insects.

Endogenous

Biochemicals which are made by and within the human body are called 'endogenous'; as opposed to exogenous, those which come from outside. For example, estradiol is an endogenous estrogen, while any phytoestrogen or pharmaceutical estrogen would be considered exogenous. Exogenous estrogens are also known as xenoestrogens; this designation includes both beneficial phytoestrogens and harmful estrogenic chemical pollutants such as DDT.

Endonuclease

An enzyme that cleaves its nucleic acid substrate at internal sites (other than the terminal bonds) in the nucleotide sequence.

Endorphins

Endogenous opiates having morphine-like effects consisting of small polypeptides such as enkephalin and leu-enkephalin and longer polypeptides such as alpha-, ß-, and gamma-endorphins. They bind to opiate receptors in the brain. Endorphins induce analgesia when injected intraventricularly but not when administered peripherally, presumably because of their inability to cross the blood/brain barrier. The amino acid sequence of the endorphins is short enough to allow the gene sequences coding for them to be synthesized.

Endospore

A highly heat and chemical resistant dormant inclusion (spore) occurring within the substance of certain genera of bacteria, mainly Bacillus and Clostridium.

Endothelial Cells

A layer of flat cells that line the tumor blood vessel structure.

Endotoxin

A poisonous complex molecule (lipopolysaccharide) that forms an integral part of the bacterial (gram-negative bacteria) cell wall and is only released when the integrity of the wall is disturbed. Certain organisms may release endotoxins (e.g. E. coli) during biosynthesis of a recombinant DNA product, thus necessitating purification steps to ensure their removal. In water treatment, it most often refers to pyrogens.

Enhanced Documentation

Collection of Engineering, Quality Control, and Regulatory Affairs documents, which will be required for the operation, validation, maintenance, and regulatory compliance of a pharmaceutical plant.

Enhanced Documentation

Adds change control and validation to Good Engineering

Practice in the Qualification process.

Enthalpy

A thermodynamic property that indicates the total energy in a sample of dry air and water vapor, measured in Btu/lb dry air. Dry air at zero degrees Fahrenheit and atmospheric pressure is designated as zero enthalpy.

Enteric coating

A coating applied to tablets which prevents them from dissolving in the stomach, but allows them to dissolve when they reach the small intestine.

Enzyme

A protein produced be living cells capable of catalysing chemical reactions without being changed itself.

2. Any of numerous proteins or conjugated proteins produced by living organisms and functioning as complex biochemical catalysts. They not only promote reactions but also function as regulators making sure the organism does not produce too much or too little of any chemical substance. Although all enzymes are proteins, many contain additional non-protein components essential for catalytic activity. Such enzymes are termed haloenzymes. The protein part of this enzyme is termed an apoenzyme and the non-amino acid part is termed a coenzyme.

3. A type of protein (almost always) that changes, constructs, or decomposes other molecules without being changed itself. A biological catalyst. Most biochemical reactions are mediated by enzymes, which help otherwise slow reactions proceed at a biologically useful pace. Enzymes are sensitive to high temperatures and extremes of pH. For example, alliinase, the enzyme that changes alliin to allicin in Garlic, is inactivated by heat (cooking) or low pH (stomach acid).

Ephedra

The drug is the aerial parts (mainly stem) obtained from *Ephedra sinica, E. equisetina* and *E. gerardiana.*

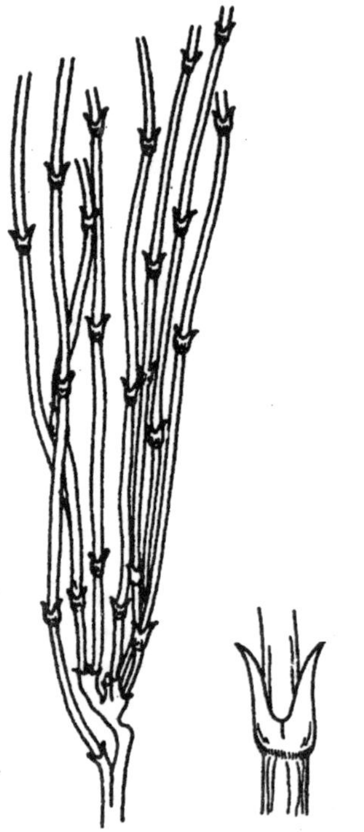

Ephedra

Epidemic

A disease attacking many people in a community simultaneously; distinguished from endemic, since the disease is not continuously present but has been introduced from outside.

Epithelium

The layer(s) of cells between an organism or its tissues or organs and their environment (skin cells, inner linings of lungs or digestive organs, outer linings of kidneys, etc.).

Epinephrine

A hormone released by the adrenal medulla in response to stimulation of the sympathetic nervous system. Also produced by tissues other than the adrenal medulla, including brain, where it functions as a neurotransmitter.

EPO (Erythropoietin)

A glycoprotein hormone that stimulates the production of red blood cells. It is a commercialized product of recombinant DNA technology.

Epoxy

These materials are based on the reactive oxirane group, which are characterized by the attachment of one oxygen atom to two different adjacent carbon atoms. Standard epoxy resins are the reaction product of bisphenol A and epichlorohydrin. Curing of epoxy resins generally occurs at ambient temperatures and is achieved by the chemical reaction of the epoxy with a second reactant such as amines, polyamines, amine products, or other reactants. Cure can occur at higher temperatures when reacted with anhydrides, carboxylic acids, phenol or novolac (phenol-formadehyde) thermoplastic resins. These reactants are sometimes referred to as catalysts, which is a misnomer.

Equine

Of, pertaining to, or characteristic of a horse, such as equine hormones.

Equipment Suitability

The established capacity of process equipment and ancillary systems to operate consistently within established limits and tolerances.

Ergot

The drug is the dried sclerotium of *Claviceps purpurea* (Fries) Tulsane.

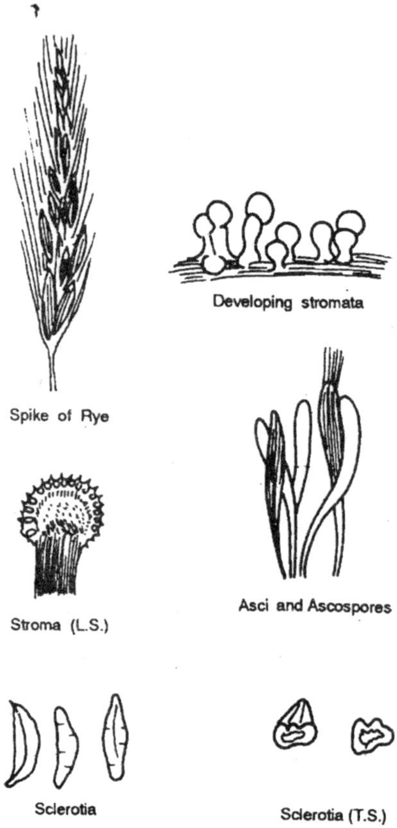

Ergot

Erythrocyte

The red blood cell consisting largely of hemoglobin and carrying nearly all the oxygen contained in the blood. Erythrocytes are biconcave discs that are manufactured in the bone marrow.

Erythromycin

An antibiotic that binds to the 50S subunit of prokaryotic

ribosomes and inhibits translocation of mRNA along the ribosome.

ESCA (Electron Spectroscopy for Chemical Analysis)

(also see: XPS (X-Ray Photoelectron Spectroscopy))

Essential Amino

Acids Amino acids that cannot be synthesized by human and other vertebrates and must be obtained from the diet.

Essential Oils

Plant products, usually somewhat volatile, giving the odours and tastes characteristic of the particular plant.

Essential Fatty Acids

The group of polyunsaturated fatty acids of plants required in the human diet.

Estrogen

Any natural or artificial substance that induces estrogenic activity; more specifically the estrogenic hormones estradiol and estrone, produced by the ovaries.

Estrogen receptor

A protein within certain cells which can bind to endogenous estrogens, phytoestrogens, or xenoestrogens. Once coupled with its estrogenic molecule, this protein communicates with other molecules and starts a process that ultimately leads to certain genes being switched on or off. The genes regulate many hormone-influenced systems.

Ethical Pharmaceutical

A controlled substance for the diagnosis or treatment of disease.

Ethylene Oxide (ETO)

A toxic compound used in gaseous form as a sterilizing agent, usually as a 10% mixture with carbon dioxide or 12% mixture with freon (referred as 12-88). Sterilization using ETO leaves residual chemicals such as ethylene chlorohydrin and ethylene glycol.

Etiologic Agent

A disease-causing organism or toxin.

Eukaryote

An organism that carries its genetic material physically constrained within a nuclear membrane, separate from the cytoplasm. All animal and plant cells except bacteria, viruses, and bluegreen algae are eukaryotic. Eukaryotes are five to ten times larger than prokaryotes in diameter.

Eutectic

Of, pertaining to, or formed at the lowest possible temperature of solidification for any mixture of specified constituents. A common term used to describe metal alloys.

Evaporator

Apparatus used in distillation to heat a liquid and create a phase change from the liquid to the vapor state. A steam boiler is an evaporator.

Excipient

A more or less inert substance added in a prescription drug compound as a diluent or vehicle or to give form or consistency when the remedy is given in a pill form; simple syrup, aromatic powder, honey, and various elixirs are examples of excipients.

Exergonic reaction

Referring to a chemical reaction that takes place with release of negative standard energy to its surroundings, a "downhill" reaction.

Exfiltration

Leakage of air out of a room through cracks in doors and pass-throughs through material transfer openings, etc. due to a difference in room pressures.

Exhaustion

Occurs when absorbents, such as activated carbon or ion exchange resins, have depleted their capacity by using up all active sites. Ion exchange resins may be regenerated to reverse the process.

Exogenous DNA

DNA originating outside an organism.

Exon

The proteincoding DNA sequence of an eukaryotic gene.

Exonuclease

An enzyme that cleaves nucleotides sequentially from free ends of a linear nucleic acid substrate.

Exotic Organism

A biological agent where either the corresponding disease does not exist in a given country or geographical area, or where the disease is the subject of prophylactic measures or an eradication program undertaken in the given country or geographical area.

Exotoxins

Proteins produced by bacteria that are able to diffuse into a medium through the bacterial cell membrane and cell wall. They are generally more potent and specific in their actions than endotoxins.

Expiration Date

The date placed on the container/labels of an API (Active Pharmaceutical Ingredient) designating the time during which the API is expected to remain within established shelf life specifications if stored under defined conditions, and after which it should not be used.

Explosion Resistance

A type of construction used to house solvents in sufficiently large quantities, to qualify the space electrically as an explosion potential area. Typically the internal walls, ceiling, and floor are constructed of material strong enough to withstand a specified intensity of explosion, and at least one wall has explosion relief devices that direct the explosion outwardly. In a single story arrangement, or if the explosion resistant area is on the top floor, the roof may also have devices that can be used to relieve the explosion.

Explosive

A chemical that causes a sudden, almost instantaneous release of pressure, gas and heat when subjected to sudden shock, pressure, or high temperatures, or a material or chemical, other than a blasting agent, that is commonly used or intended for the purpose of producing an explosive effect.

Exposed or Open Process

The drug substance is exposed to the room environment during processing.

Express

To translate the genetic information stored in the DNA into protein.

Expression System

A host organism combined with a genetic vector (such as virus or circular DNA molecule called a plasmid) that is loaded with a gene of interest. The expression system provides the genetic context in which a gene will function in the cell - that is, the gene will be expressed as a protein.

Extract

A concentrated form of natural substance obtained by treating crude materials containing these substances with a solvent. Extracts are classed as solid extracts, fluid extracts, liquid extracts, powdered extracts, tinctures, and native extracts.

Extractables

Undesirable foreign substances that are leached or dissolved by water or process streams from the materials of construction used in filters, storage vessels, distribution piping, and other wetted surfaces.

F

Face Velocity

The velocity obtained by dividing the air quantity by the component face area (NEBB).

Facility Flexibility

A qualitative measure of the number of different products that can be produced in a facility or area of a facility.

Facility User

The end user of a facility, often called the Owner, represented by operating, maintenance, and quality control personnel.

Factor VIII (Hemophilia Factor)

Also known as antihemophilic factor or AHF (Brinkhous) in the clotting of blood, Factor VIII is a labile protein of the blood-clotting system that assists in the conversion of Factor IX into plasma factor X (Stuart factor). Deficiency of factor VIII is associated with classic hemophilia A, a hereditary, sex-linked, hemorrhagic tendency that occurs almost exclusively in men; clotting time is prolonged, less thromboplastin is formed, and the conversion of prothrombin is diminished.

Factor IX (Hemophilia Factor)

In the clotting of blood, also known as Christmas factor (Biggs and Macfarlane). Deficiency of factor IX causes hemophilia B or Christmas disease that resembles hemophilia A, and is an inherited defect that leads to a severe hemorrhagic disorder. Factor IX is required for the formation of intrinsic blood thromboplastin and affects the amount formed (rather than the rate).

False unicorn (Chamaelirium luteum)

Balances hormones; diuretic; aids in delayed or absent menstruation; also helps threatened miscarriage; in small dosages it eases vomiting associated with pregnancy.

FDA Form 483

The official form of notification prepared at the conclusion of an inspection (without review by FDA management) listing observations of perceived violations of Good Manufacturing Practices that may constitute violations of law in the opinion of an inspector. Originally intended to inform companies of possible product adulteration, they must be replied to satisfactorily and/or corrective action taken in order to alleviate any offensive notification and avoid action from the FDA (i.e., plant shut-down). Accessible through the Freedom of Information Act to competitors, potential customers, and the media; 483s can lead to withholding of product approvals, may come into play in due diligence phases of acquisitions and mergers, and can potentially cost companies money.

Fed-Batch Fermentation

The most common operating mode for rDNA fermentation. After an initial partial charge of media to the fermenter and seed transfer, sterile media is added at measured rates during the balance of the fermentation cycle. Cell mass and broth are withdrawn only at the end of the cycle.

Federal Standard 209E

The document that established standard classes of air cleanliness for airborne particulate levels in cleanrooms and clean zones. It prescribed methods for classes of air cleanliness for airborne particulate levels in cleanrooms and clean zones. It prescribed methods for class verification and monitoring of air cleanliness. It also addressed certain other factors but only as they affected control of airborne particulate contamination.

Federal Standard 209E is in the process of being replaced by ISO 14644-1.

Feedback Loop

A central concept in industrial controls in which the value of a process variable is compared with the desired value (setpoint), and any discrepancy (error) is converted into a modified output signal.

Feedwater

The water entering a treatment process.

Fennel

Fennel *(Foeniculum vulgare)* is a plant of the Apiaceae or parsley family, which produces edible seeds and leaves. The variety Florence fennel *(F. vulgare azoricum)* has inflated leaf bases which form a sort of bulb. It comes mainly from India and Egypt and it has an anise-like flavor, but is more aromatic and sweeter. Its flavor comes from anethole, an aromatic compound that also flavors anise and star anise.

It is a perennial herb, erect, glaucous, and grows to 2 m tall. It is highly aromatic. The leaves grow up to 40 cm long; they are finely dissected, with the ultimate segments filiform; umbels are terminal, 5-15 cm wide; umbellets with 20-50 tiny flowers, these are on filiform pedicels. The fruit is from 4-9 mm long, half as wide or less, and grooved.

Florence fennel is much smaller than the wild type and has inflated leaf bases which are eaten as a vegetable, both raw and cooked. There are several cultivars of Florence fennel, which is also known by several other names, notably finocchio. Fennel is native to southern Europe (especially by the Mediterranean) and southwestern Asia. In Hawaii, it is cultivated and naturalized along roadsides, in pastures, and other open sites. It has been similarly widely introduced to the US and southern Canada. In Fiji, it is occasionally cultivated near sea level, and sparingly naturalized in shady waste places. It is propagated by seed.

It is used traditionally as a leaf vegetable or herb in cooking, particularly with eggs and fish. It is also used as a diuretic and to improve milk supply of breastfeeding mothers.

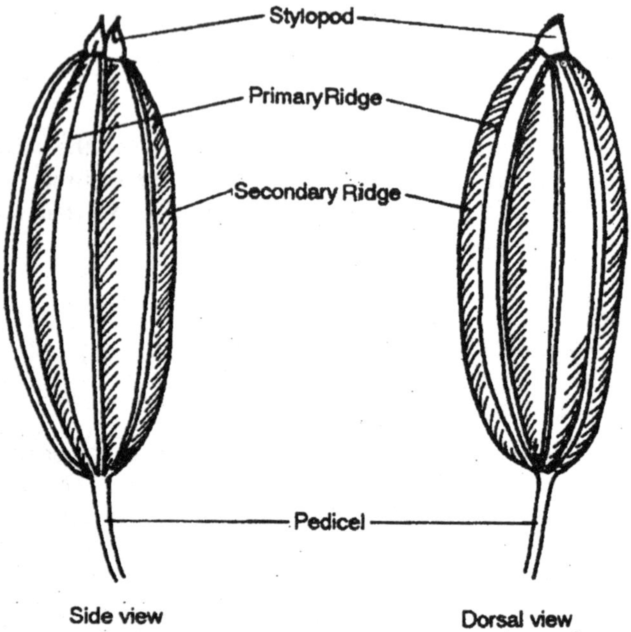

Fennel

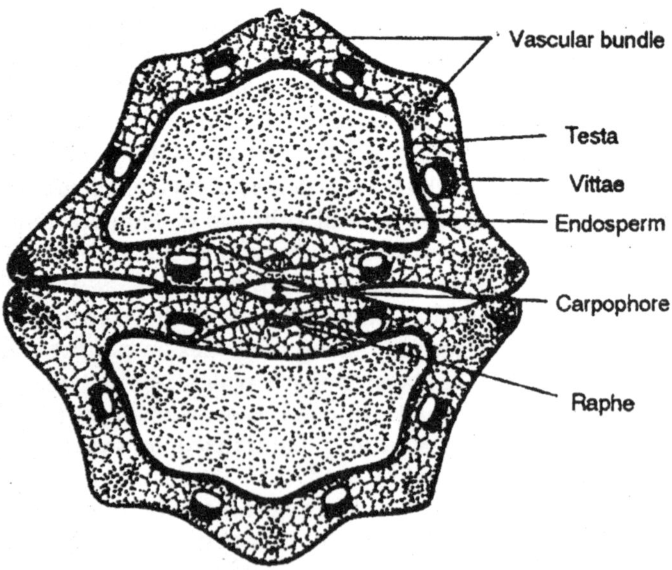

Fennel

Florence fennel, popular in Italy and Germany, among other countries, may be eaten as a salad (e.g. with chicory and avocado), blanched and marinated, or cooked (e.g. as risotto); in all cases, it adds its characteristic mild anise flavor.

Many Indian restaurants will have a dish of fennel seed with small candies mixed therein near the entrance. Some patrons of these establishments will eat a spoonful on their way out as a digestive and to cleanse the palate.

Fennel is also used in some natural toothpastes.

Braised Fennel

Ingredients

1 Fennel bulb Half pint of vegetable stock 1 Clove of Garlic Sunflower or olive oil

Get a metal based saucepan and heat the oil. Meanwhile cut the tops off the fennel bulb so that you are left with only the bulbous part. Now cut it into quarters and fry each side of the pieces in the oil until lightly browned.

Crush and chop the garlic and mix it in with the stock. Now pour the stock into the saucepan and boil until it reduces to become a coating sauce.

Serve with some steamed vegetables and a smile.

In Ancient Greek fennel was called marathron. This is the origin of the placename Marathon (meaning place of fennel), site of the Battle of Marathon in 490 BC.

In medieval times fennel was used in conjunction with St Johns Wort to keep away witchcraft and other evil things. Personally I think that this might have originated for the fact that it can be used as an insect repellant.

Fennel is thought to be one of the nine herbs held sacred by the Anglo-saxons the others are still not totally certain but they seem to be Mugwort (Artemisia vulgaris), Greater Plantain (Plantago major), Watercress (Nastrurtium officinale), Wild Chamomile (Matricaria recutita), Stinging Nettle (Urtica dioica), Crab Apple (pyrus malus) , Chervil (Anthriscus cerefolium) and Viper's Bugloss (Echium vulgare) the final one still remains a mystery.

An estrogenic agent38; a lactagogue.

Fenugreek

Fenugreek, also called **methi**, is a crop plant grown as a potherb and for the spice made from its seeds. The fenugreek plant grows wild from the eastern Mediterranean area to China; it is cultivated worldwide.

A side effect of consuming even small amounts of fenugreek is a maple syrup or curry smell in the eater's sweat and urine which is caused by the potent aroma compound sotolone. Fenugreek is frequently used in the production of flavoring for artificial syrups. The taste of toasted fenugreek is additionally based on substituted pyrazines, as is cumin. By itself, it has a somewhat bitter taste.

Fenugreek is one of the spices frequently used in the preparation of curry powders and pastes, and is often encountered in the cuisine of India and Thailand. The young leaves and sprouts of fenugreek are eaten as greens and the fresh or dried leaves are used to flavor other dishes. Fenugreek is also one of four herbs used for the Iranian recipe Ghormeh Sabzi.

Fenugreek seed is widely used as a galactagogue (milk producing agent) by nursing mothers to increase inadequate breast milk supply. It can be found in capsule form in many health food stores.

The name fenugreek or *foenum-graecum* is from Latin for "Greek hay".

Fermentation

The process of growing microorganisms within an enclosed tank (fermenter) under controlled conditions of aeration, agitation, temperature, and pH. The different types organisms used as a basis for fermentation are:

1. Bacteria (E. coli)
2. Yeasts
3. Molds
4. Chinese Hamster Ovary (CHO) cells
5. Kidney cells
6. Vaccines to viruses

Fermentation

The biochemical synthesis of organic compounds by microorganisms.

Fermenter

A tank or vessel used for carrying out fermentation. There are

various choices of fermenters, depending on whether cells are suspended in the medium or attached to some type of support:
1. In suspension reactors
2. Attached growth reactors
3. Stirred-tank reactors
4. Airlift fermenters
5. Packed bed reactors
6. Two-chamber reactors
7. Hollow-fiber reactors
Fetal Calf Serum
The liquid portion remaining after natural coagulation of blood drawn from the heart of an unborn calf. Because of the absence of gamma globulin, fetal calf serum is a good tissue culture serum.

Fever

Also known as pyrexia, a human body temperature above the normal 98.6°F (37°C).
Fiber Any particulate contaminant having an aspect (length to width) ratio of 10 or more.

Feverfew (Tanateum parsenium)

Anti-inflammatory for arthritis; remedy for migraine headaches; relieves painful and slow menstrual flows; promotes relaxation; uterine stimulant.

Fibrin

A whitish, filamentous protein formed by the action of thrombin or fibrinogen. The conversion of fibrinogen, a hydrosol, into fibrin, a hydro gel, is the basis for the clotting of blood.
2. A plasma protein that, in its aggregated state, is the major component of a blood clot. It is produced from fibrinogen, a soluble precursor, by the action of the proteolytic enzyme, thrombin.

Fibrinogen

In the clotting of blood it is known as Factor I. The plasma protein that becomes converted to a clot at the end of the coagulation process. Present in plasma; absent in serum.

Fibroblast

Any cell or corpuscle from which connective tissue is developed. syn: desmocyte; fibrocyte.

Filé powder

Filé powder, also called **gumbo filé,** is used in the making of gumbo, a thick Cajun soup. Together with okra, it provides the distinctive flavor and texture of the soup.

Traditionally, filé powder is made from sassafras, which has been shown to cause liver cancer in laboratory studies [1]. For this reason, major grocery-store spice brands sell a mixture of other herbs as filé powder. Genunine sassafras is available from specialty suppliers, who claim that the health risks are negligible when ordinary amounts of filé powder is used.

Filé powder has also been made traditionally from Sassafras leaves, which do not contain safrole, the volatile oil linked with cancer in lab rats. Filé powder made from sassafras leaves can still be found commercially and is used extensively in Louisiana.

Filtration

Removal of suspended matter from a fluid by passing it through a porous matrix that prevents particles from getting through, usually by entrapment on or in the filter matrix.

Fill and Finish (Parenteral Drugs)

Preparation of parenteral drugs, either LVPs or SVPs, demands the highest level of contamination control, because the human body's normal defenses against infection are bypassed when parenteral medications are introduced either intramuscularly (I.M.) or intravenously (I.V.) directly into the body. The processing of raw materials into finished dosage forms must comply at all times with cGMPs and must be able to support process validation. Mechanical design should include HVAC Classifications considered essential to attain global regulatory acceptance. For classifications, see the ISPE® Guide for Sterile Manufacturing Facilities. The desire for increased levels of sterility assurance has led the FDA to promote the use of terminal sterilization for asepticaliy filled products. The FDA has stated that terminal sterilization processing is the method of choice unless the manufacturer can show that it is detrimental to the product. Terminal sterilization may be accomplished using autoclaves that apply overpressure to balance the pressures that are developed across the inside and outside of the containers. Because of product sensitivities, biologics, and blood products are not appropriate applications for terminal sterilization.

Final Bulk Product

The final drug product after chemical or biological processing and purification, ready for concentration, drying, and filling into containers prior to dispensing and final filling.

Finished Product

A medicinal product that has undergone all stages of production, including packaging in its final container.

Firmware

A combination of hardware and software with the programming written directly into read-only memory (ROM).

FISH (Fluorescent In Situ Hybridization)

A physical mapping approach that uses fluorescein tags to detect hybridization of probes with metaphase chromosomes and with the less condensed somatic interface chromatin.

Fissile Material

A radioisotope that could undergo a nuclear fission reaction and is usually found at reactor sites or as part of a nuclear weapon.

Flaggelae

Thin, helical filaments attached to the surface of bacterial and eukaryotic (e.g. sperm, protozoa) cells. They are motile structures containing microtubules (composed of proteins called tubulin) that enable cells possessing them to move.

Flammable Liquid

A liquid having a closed cup flash point below 100°F (37.8°C).

Flammable liquids do not include compressed gases or cryogenic fluids. Flammable liquids are subdivided as follows: 1. Class I-A - Liquids having a closed cup flash point below 73°F (22.8°C) and having a boiling point below 100°F (37.8°C). 2. Class I-B - liquids having a closed cup flash point below 73°F (22.8°C) and having a boiling point at or above 100°F (37.8°C). 3. Class I-C - liquids having a closed cup flash point at or above 73°F (22.8°C) and below 100°F (37.8°C).

Flammable Solid

A solid substance, other than one which is defined as a blasting agent or explosive, that is liable to cause fire through friction or as a result of retained heat from manufacture, which has an ignition temperature below 212°F (100°C), or which burns so vigorously or persistently when ignited that it creates a serious hazard. Flammable solids include finely divided solid materials which when dispersed in air as a cloud could be ignited and cause an explosion.

Flaws

Metallic flaws are unintentional irregularities that occur at one place or at relatively infrequent or widely varying intervals on the surface. Flaws include such defects such as cracks, blowholes, inclusions, pits, checks, ridges, scratches, and other surface abnormalities.

Floc

Mass having a fluffy or wooly appearance.

Flocculation

A technique for liquid/solids separation. Cationic or anionic polyelectrolytes (e.g. polyacrylamides) are added to highly colloidal water causing coagulation and subsequent settling. The phenomena could be charge neutralization or a bridging effect between separate particles.

Flow Cytometry

Analysis of biological material by detection of light-absorbing or fluorescing properties of cells or subcellular fractions (i.e., chromosomes) passing in a narrow stream through a laser beam. An absorbance or fluorescence profile of the sample is produced. Automated sorting devices, used to fractionate samples, sort successive droplets of the analyzed stream into different fractions depending on the fluorescence emitted by each droplet.

Flow Decay

Measuring the decline in flow rate through a filter to establish a Silt Index for the water being filtered. The Silt Index is a measure of suspended solids and their ability to clog the filter.

Flow Restrictor

A flow-limiting orifice used to control flow rate or pressure drop in a liquid stream.

Fluid extract

Solution of the soluble constituents of vegetable drugs such that each millilitre represents one gram of the drug. Fluid extracts contain alcohol as both solvent and a preservative.

Fluid Service (piping)

As defined in ASME B31.3, fluid service is a general term concerning the application of a piping system, considering the combination of fluid properties, operating conditions, and other factors, which establish the basis for design of the piping system.

1. Category D Fluid Service: A fluid service in which all the following apply: (a) the fluid handled is nonflammable, nontoxic, and not damaging to human tissues (see definition below). (b) The design gage pressure does not exceed 1035 kPA (150 psi). (c) The design temperature is from -29°C (-20°F) through 186°C (366°F).

2. Category M Fluid Service: A fluid service in which the potential for personnel exposure is judged to be significant and in which a single exposure to a very small quantity of a toxic fluid, caused by leakage can produce serious irreversible harm to persons upon breathing or bodily contact, even when prompt restorative measures are taken.

3. High Pressure Fluid Service: A fluid service for which the

owner specifies the use of chapter IX (High Pressure Piping) for piping design and construction.

4. Normal Fluid Service: A fluid service pertaining to most piping covered by ASME B31.3, i.e., not subject to the rules for Category D, Category M, or High Pressure Fluid Service, and not subject to severe cyclic conditions.

Damaging to human tissues for the purpose of the Code, describes a fluid service in which exposure to the fluid, caused by leakage under expected operating conditions, can harm skin, eyes, or exposed mucous membranes so that irreversible damage may result unless prompt restorative measures are taken. These measures may include, flushing with water, administration of antidotes, or medication.

Fluidized Bed

A container holding powder coating material which is aerated from below so as to form an air-supported expanded cloud of such material through which the preheated object to be coated is immersed and transported.

Fluorescein

An orange-red compound, C20H12O5, which exhibits intense fluorescence in alkaline solution.

Fluorinated Plastics

Fluorinated plastics are thermoplastic paraffinic polymers where the hydrogen has been replaced by fluorine, and in some cases, chlorine. These materials are some of the more popular in the CPI because of good chemical resistance to a wide variety of aggressive chemicals, and relatively high heat resistance of 400°F to 500°F. They include FEP, PTFE, PFA, PCTFE, ETFE, PVDF, and PVF.

Flux Removers

Chlorinated solvents with alcohols that may be sprayed from aerosol cans to remove welding flux.

Follicle stimulating hormone (FSH)

Hormone produced by the anterior pituitary. FSH stimulates growth of the follicle in the ovaries and spermatogenesis in the testes.

Forest Management

Strategy, in theory, that reconciles the economic interests of producers with the needs of conservation.

Formaldehyde

A colorless, highly irritating, pungent compound used in the pharmaceutical and cosmetic industries as an antimicrobial agent.

Forward Flow Test

An objective and quantitative method of determining filter integrity. A test in which the filter is wetted and a predetermined constant air pressure is applied. A measurement of pure diffusional airflow through the wetted membrane is made. If the diffusional airflow across the membrane is below the maximum allowable value given, then the filter is acceptable.

Fouling

Occurs when gelatinous coatings, colloidal masses, or dense bacterial growth form a compacted crust on membrane or filter surfaces which blocks further flow.

Food Chain

The trophic interrelationship of species within an ecosystem.

Free radicals

A molecule containing an odd number of electrons; free radicals contain an open bond or a half bond and are highly reactive. 2. A free radical is an 'oxidant,' 'oxidizer' or 'oxidizing agent,' a molecule with one 'extra' electron that wants to take an electron away from another molecule and use that electron to stabilize itself (electrons are happiest in pairs). This process damages ('oxidizes') many biological chemicals including the lipids in cell membranes.

Freeze drying

Plant materials are frozen, then subject to high vacuum. Water molecules sublimate (pass from solid to gas phase), and are removed from the material. The drying is all done at low temperature.

Fruit

Fruits may be simple (developed from single carpel) or aggregate (formed from many carpels). They may be further dry (coriander, fennel) or fleshy (organge, lemon).

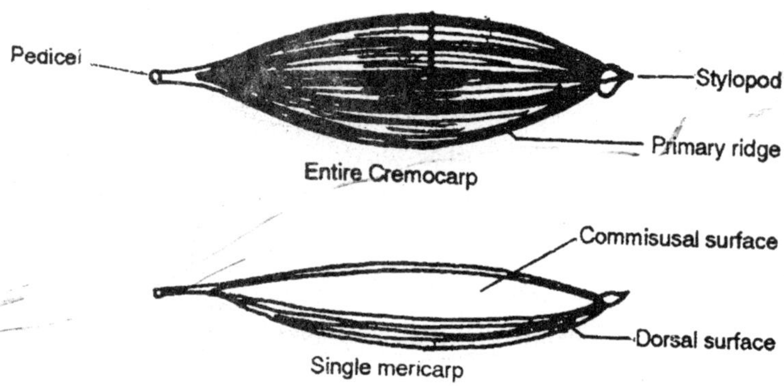

Cremocarp

Fume Hoods

Units that collect fumes from chemicals, solvents, acids, and other hazardous materials. Hoods may include HEPA filters if powders are present, or carbon filters to filter fumes from the work surface and return cleaned air to the room. Most fume hoods are 100% exhausted to outdoors. A glass, Plexiglas™ or acrylic front panel may be included for worker safety.

Functional Description A written description of what a system is to do with sequence of operation relating activities to Critical Parameters (Why the system does what it does for GMP reasons). A non-GMP system should also have a functional specification to aid designers and software development.

Functional Gene Tests

Biochemical assays for a specific protein, which indicates that a specific gene is not merely present but active.

Functional group

In organic molecules, particular groups of atoms where

characteristic chemical reactions take place. There is a limited number of functional groups, and they can be found in many different kinds of molecules. Examples: Alcohol group, -OH; Amine group, $-NH_2$; Sulfide group, C-S-C.

Functionality

Suitability for the intended purpose.

Fungi

Plural of fungus. Low forms of plant life unable to form protein and carbohydrates (heterotrophs) that are widespread in nature. Fungal cells are larger than bacterial cells, and their typical internal structures, such as nucleus and vacuoles, can be seen easily with a light microscope. On the basis of their mode of sexual reproduction, fungi are grouped in four classes: Phycomycetes, Ascomycetes, Deuteromycetes (Fungi Imperfectii), and Basidiomycetes. Two major groups of fungi are the yeasts and molds. (also see: Mycelium)
Fungicide An agent that destroys fungi.

Fusion

The melting together of filler metal and base metal, or of base metal only, that results in coalescence.

Fusion Welding

Welding in which the base material is fused together without the addition of filler material to the weld.

G

Gaia hypothesis

Postulates that the earth behaves like a living organism with living things and the environment evolving together..each affecting the other.

Galangal

Galangal, is a root with culinary and medicinal uses, best known in the west today for its appearance in Thai cuisine (e.g., *Tom kha gai*) but also common in recipes from medieval Europe. It resembles ginger in appearance and taste but has an extra citrus aroma with a slight hint of soapiness. It is available as a powder from vendors of Oriental spices and also available in whole, cut or powdered from vendors of herbs. Also known as Galingale or Laos (its Indonesian name). Coincidentally, it is one of the most prominent herbs in Lao cuisine.

The word galangal, or its variant galanga is used as a common name for all members of the genus Alpinia, but in common usage can refer to four plants, all in the Zingiberaceae:

- *Alpinia galanga* or Greater galangal
- *Alpinia officinarum* or Lesser galangal
- *Kaempferia galanga,* also called **Lesser galangal** or **Sand ginger**
- *Boesenbergia pandurata,* also called **Chinese ginger** or fingerroot

A. galanga is also known as Chewing John, Little John Chew

and Galanga Root. Under these names, it is used in folk medicine and in voodoo charms.

Gamete

Mature male or female reproductive cell (sperm or ovum) with a haploid set of chromosomes (23 for humans).

Gamma-amino butyric acid (GABA)

An amino acid, which functions as an inhibitory neurotransmitter in the central nervous system.

Gamma Globulin

A blood protein that plays a major role in the process of immunity. Sometimes the term "gamma globulin" refers to a whole group of blood proteins that are known as antibodies or immunoglobulins (Ig). Most often, however, it applies to a particular immunoglobulin, designated as IgG, believed to be the most abundant type of antibody in the body.

Garlic

Garlic (Allium sativum) is a bulbous perennial food plant of the family Alliaceae. The word comes to us from Old English garleac, meaning "spear leek".

Because of its wide cultivation, its origins are uncertain; it has been traced to both southwest Siberia and Sicily, where it grows wild. It is related to onions and lilies. The domesticated garlic plant does not produce seeds, but is grown from bulbs. These bulbs, whose segments are usually called "cloves" by cooks, are the part of the plant most commonly eaten, though some cooks also use the early spring shoots. These shoots are often pickled in Russia and states of the Caucasus and eaten as an appetizer.

(A common error of beginning cooks is to misinterpret the word "clove" as meaning the entire garlic bulb, rather than one of its segments, thereby wildly exaggerating the amount of garlic in a recipe.)

Garlic is most often used as a seasoning or a condiment, and is believed to have some medicinal value, notably against hypertension. When crushed or finely chopped it yields allicin, a powerful antibiotic and anti-fungal compound. It also contains alliin, ajoene, enzymes, vitamin B, minerals, and flavonoids.

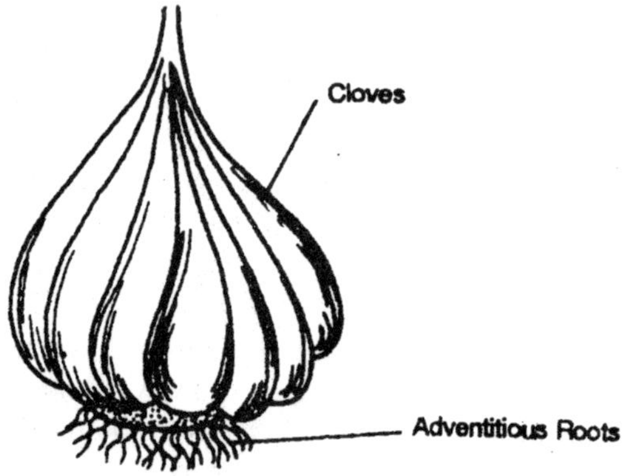

Garlic

It has long, narrow, flat, obscurely keeled leaves, a deciduous spathe, and a globose umbel of whitish flowers, among which are small bulbils. The bulb has membranous scales, in the axils of which are 10 or 12 cloves, or smaller bulbs. From these new bulbs can be procured by planting out in late winter or early spring.

The bulbs are best preserved hung in a dry place. If of fair size, four to six of them weigh about 1 lb (0.5 kg). To prevent the plant from running to leaf, Pliny (Nat. Hist. xix. 34) advised bending the stalk downward and covering with earth; seeding, he observes, may be prevented by twisting the stalk. (By "seeding", he mostly likely means the development of small, less potent bulbs.)

Garlic is cultivated in the same manner as the shallot. It is stated to have been grown in England before the year 1548. The percentage composition of the bulbs is as water 84.09, organic matter 13.38, and inorganic matter 1.53—that of the leaves being water 87.14, organic matter 11.27 and inorganic matter 1.59.

The bulb has a strong and characteristic odor and an acrid taste, and yields an offensively smelling oil, essence of garlic, identical with allyl sulphide ($C_6H_{10}S_2$). This, when garlic has been eaten, is evolved by the excretory organs, the activity of which it promotes. When eaten in quantity, garlic may be strongly evident in the diner's sweat the following day. The well-known phenomenon of "garlic breath" can be alleviated by eating fresh parsley and this is included in many garlic recipes. Because of its strong odor, garlic is sometimes called the "stinking rose".

From the earliest times garlic has been used as an article of diet. It formed part of the food of the Israelites in Egypt (Numb. xi. 5) and of the labourers employed by Cheops in the construction of his pyramid. Garlic is still grown in Egypt, where, however, the Syrian is the kind most esteemed (see Rawlinson's Herodotus, 2.125).

It was largely consumed by the ancient Greek and Roman soldiers, sailors and rural classes (cf. Virg. Ed. ii. II), and, as Pliny tells us (N.H. xix. 32), by the African peasantry. Galen eulogizes it as the "rustic's theriac" (cure-all), and Alexander Neckam, a writer of the 12th century, recommends it as a palliative of the heat of the sun in field labor.

"The people in places where the simoon is frequent," says Mountstuart Elphinstone, "eat garlic, and rub their lips and noses with it, when they go out in the heat of the summer, to prevent their suffering by the simoon." "O dura messorum ilia," exclaims Horace (Epod. iii.), as he records his detestation of the popular esculent, to smell of which was accounted a sign of vulgarity (cf. Shakespeare, Coriol. iv. 6, and Meas. for Meas. Iii. 2).

Garlic was rare in traditional English cuisine, and a much more common ingredient in southern Europe. Garlic was placed by the ancient Greeks on the piles of stones at cross-roads, as a supper for Hecate (Theophrastus, Characters, l~.eunbcuuoviac); and according to Pliny garlic and onions were invoked as deities by the Egyptians at the taking of oaths. The inhabitants of Pelusium in lower Egypt, who worshipped the onion, are said to have held both it and garlic in aversion as food. Garlic possesses stimulant and stomachic properties, and was of old, as still sometimes now, employed as a medicinal remedy.

Pliny (N.H. xx. 23) gives an exceedingly long list of complaints in which it was considered beneficial. Dr T Sydenham valued it as an application in confluent smallpox, and, says Cullen (Mat. Med. ii. p. 174, 1789), found some dropsies cured by it alone. Early in the 20th century, it was sometimes used in the treatment of pulmonary tuberculosis or phthisis.

In the United States, Gilroy, California promotes itself as "Garlic Capital of the World."

The wild "crow garlic" and "field garlic" of Britain are the species Allium vineale and A. oleraceum, respectively.

The term "wild garlic" is now used to refer to ramsons (Allium ursinum). In North America, "wild garlic" or "crow garlic" is (Allium vineale), and along with "wild onion" (also known as "meadow garlic" or "wild garlic") (Allium canada) are common weeds in fields.

Classification of culinary garlic can be complex. The broadest division is into "hardneck" and "softneck" types; very broadly speaking, hardnecks have more intense flavors—they are more closely related to their wild ancestor—but lesser storage capabilities, while conversely softnecks are excellent "keepers" but often milder (those are broad-brush simplifications with numerous exceptions and half-exceptions.) Within those two types, there are usually felt to be three subdivisions of hardnecks and two of softnecks. One scheme, with some flavor notes from a commercial grower, is this:

- Hardneck:
    - Rocambole - rich, full-bodied flavor
    - Porcelain - much like rocambole
    - Purple Stripe - these often win "baked-garlic" taste tests:
        - Purple Stripe per se
        - Glazed Purple Stripe
        - Marbled Purple Stripe
- Softneck:
    - Artichoke - "milder" flavors:
        - Artichoke per se
        - Asiatic
        - Turban
    - Silverskin:
        - Silverskin per se - the familiar supermarket garlic
        - Creole

The types differ not only in culinary qualities, but in storage potential. Under good storage conditions, which are not hard to achieve (room temperature and medium to low humidity), one can hope for these results:

- Asiatic and Turban types: a few months
- Rocambole and Purple Stripe types: 6 months
- Porcelain and Artichoke types: 8 to 10 months
- Silverskin (including Creole) types: up to a full year

Rocamboles, however, have a tendency to dehydrate in storage under dry conditions (less than about 50% humidity).

This article incorporates text from the public domain 1911 Encyclopædia Britannica.

Plant the individual cloves from a garlic plant in drills of 5cm (2inches) and 15cm (6 inches) apart. Ideal soil pH is in the 6.2 to 6.8 range. Garlic grows best in hot wet conditions, but try it all year round. It is pretty hardy and will live through frosts. Ensure that the growing area is weed free. Garlic likes water, in a hot climate it may need to be watered daily. If the shoots look dry then it is a sign that the plant needs a 'drink'.

Garlic is ready to harvest in about four months after it has been sown at this point the foilage will loose its colour and die back .Dig up with a fork to avoid damaging the bulbs.

Garlic is claimed by some to have many significant medicinal benefits, but there has been no demonstration of the effects of garlic that meets commonly accepted scientific standards.

The cloves are used by aficionados for infections, especially chest problems, digestive disorders, and fungal infections such as thrush. They are claimed to be an effective long-term remedy for cardiovascular problems reducing excessive blood cholesteral levels, atherosclerosis, the risk of thrombosis, and hypertension but these claims are disputed as there has been no clinical trial that has demonstrated any such benefits. Garlic is also alleged to help regulate blood sugar levels, and so can be helpful in late-onset diabetes, though people taking insulin should not consume medicinal amounts of garlic without consulting a physician. Best used fresh.

Lowers blood pressure and cholesterol level39; increases phagocyte and peritoneal macrophage production, thereby acting as an antimicrobial; effective in treating throat infection40.

Gas Metal Arc Welding (GMAW)

An arc welding process that produces coalescence of metals by heating them with an arc between a continuous filler metal (consumable) electrode and the work. Shielding is obtained entirely from an externally supplied gas or gas mixture. Some variations of this process are called MIG (Metal Inert Gas) Or CO2 welding, nonpreferred terms.

Gas Room

A separately ventilated, fully enclosed room in which only toxic and highly toxic compressed gases and associated equipment and supplies are stored or used.

Gas Tungsten Arc Welding (GTAW)

An arc welding process that produces coalescence of metals by heating them with an arc between a tungsten (nonconsumable) electrode and the work. Shielding is obtained from a gas or gas mixture. Pressure may or may not be used and filler material may or may not be used. (This process is sometimes called TIG (Tungsten Inert Gas) welding, a nonpreferred term).

Gel

A colloid, where the dispersed phase is liquid and the dispersion medium is solid.

Gel Electrophoresis

A DNA separation technique that is very important in DNA sequencing. Standard sequencing procedures involve cloning DNA fragments into special sequencing cloning vectors that carry tiny pieces of DNA. The next step is to determine the base sequence of the tiny fragments by a special procedure that generates a series of even tinier DNA fragments that differ in size by only one base. These nested fragments are separated by gel electrophoresis, in which the DNA pieces are added to a gelatinous solution, allowing the fragments to work their way down through the gel. Smaller pieces move faster and will reach the bottom first. Movement through the gel is hastened by applying an electrical field to the gel.

Gel Polarization

The phenomenon of formation of a layer of insoluble/semi-soluble material at a liquid/filter interface. It is a common occurrence with excessive linear velocity flow through filters of colloidal suspensions and macromolecular solutions.

Gelatin

A derived protein formed from the collagen of the tissues by boiling in water, sometimes called an albuminoid, though it lacks the characteristic albuminoid properties. Glue, size, and isinglass are forms of gelatin.

Gene

A natural unit of hereditary material that is the physical basis for the transmission of the characteristics of living organisms from one generation to another. The basic genetic material is fundamentally the same in all living organisms. It consists of deoxyribonucleic acid (DNA) in most organisms and ribonucleic acid (RNA) in certain viruses, and is usually associated in a linear arrangement that, in part, constitutes the chromosome. The average length of a gene is 1μm and thus, about one million genes could be contained in a one-meter stretch of DNA. The segment of DNA that is involved in producing a polypeptide chain, it includes regions preceding (leader) and following (trailer) the coding region as well as intervening sequences (introns) between individual coding segments (exons).

Gene Expression

The process by which a gene's coded information is converted into the structures present and operating in the cell. Expressed genes include those that are transcribed into mRNA and then translated into protein and those that are transcribed into RNA but not translated into protein.

Gene Family

Group of closely related genes that makes similar products.

Gene Mapping

Determination of the relative positions of genes on a DNA

molecule (chromosome or plasmid) and of the distance, in linkage units or physical units, between them.

Gene Markers

Landmarks for a target gene, either detectable traits that are inherited along with the gene, or distinctive segments of DNA.

Gene Product

The biochemical material, either RNA or protein, resulting from expression of a gene. The amount of gene product is used to measure how active a gene is; abnormal amounts can be correlated with disease causing alleles.

Gene Sequencing

The determination of the sequence of bases in a DNA strand. The two most widely used methods are the chain-termination method, developed by Sanger in the mid-seventies, and the chemical method developed by Maxam & Gilbert around the same time.

Gene Splicing

The enzymatic attachment of one gene or part of a gene to another.

Gene Therapy

The insertion of normal DNA directly into cells to correct a generic defect.

Generic Drug

A drug produced and marketed under its chemical or "generic" name (e.g. acetaminophen) as opposed to "Tylenol", a brand name for the former produced by Johnson & Johnson. A generic drug can be sold only after a proprietary drug goes off patent (i.e. when the patent runs out after 17 years). There are numerous generic drug manufacturers. While generic drugs are cheaper for consumers, they still must meet the standards of GMPs as set out by the FDA.

Genetics

The scientific study of heredity: how particular qualities or traits are transmitted from parents to offspring.

Genetic Code

The sequence of nucleotides, coded in triplets (codons) along the mRNA that determines the sequence of amino acids in protein synthesis. The DNA sequence of a gene can be used to predict the mRNA sequence, and the genetic code can in turn be used to predict the amino acid sequence.

Genetic Diseases

Diseases that occur because a mutation in the genetic material.

Genetic Engineering

The selective, deliberate alteration of genes by technological means.

Genome Project

Research and technology development effort aimed at mapping and sequencing some or all of the genome human beings and other organisms.

Genomic Library

A collection of clones made from a set of randomly generated overlapping DNA fragments representing the entire genome of an organism.

Genomic Sequence

The order of the subunits, called bases, that makes up a particular fragment of DNA in a genome. DNA is a long molecule made up of four different kinds of bases, which are abbreviated A, C, T, and G. A DNA fragment that is 10 bases long might have a base sequence of, for example, ATCGTTCCTG. The particular sequence of bases encodes important information in an individual's genetic blueprint, and is unique for each individual (except identical twins).

Genotype

The genetic composition of an organism (including expressed and nonexpressed genes), which may not be readily apparent.

Gentian (Gentiana lutea)

Increases ability to digest and assimilate food41; increases sensitivity of glands and organs to adrenalin (the hormone the body secretes when in need of rapid energy)42.

Germicidal Lamps

Light sources that emit ultraviolet radiation at a wavelength of 254 nanometers. These lights are commonly found in biological safety cabinets and used to inactivate bacteria, viruses and fungi which are either airborne or on exposed surfaces.

Germicide

An agent that destroys microorganisms, especially pathogenic microorganisms ("germs"). Sterilants, disinfectants, and antiseptics are germicides.

Germplasm

The total genetic variability, represented by germ cells or seeds, available to a particular population of organisms.

Ginger

Ginger root is used extensively as a spice in many if not most cuisines of the world. Though called a root, it is actually the rhizome of the monocotyledonous plant Zingiber officinale. The active constituent of giner is zingerone.

Young ginger roots are juicy and fleshy with a very mild taste. They are often pickled in vinegar or sherry as a snack or just cooked as an ingredient in many dishes. Mature ginger roots are fibrous and nearly dry. The juice from old ginger roots is extremely potent and is often used as a spice in Chinese cuisine to cover up other strong odors and flavors such as in seafood and mutton.

Ginger is also made into candy, is used as a flavoring for cookies and cake, and is the main flavor in ginger ale, a sweet, carbonated, non-alcoholic beverage.

In Western cuisine, ginger is traditionally restricted to sweet foods, such as ginger ale, gingerbread, and ginger snaps (a type of cookie).

Powdered dry ginger is used to add spiciness to gingerbread and other recipes. It tastes quite different from fresh ginger, and neither can be substituted for the other.

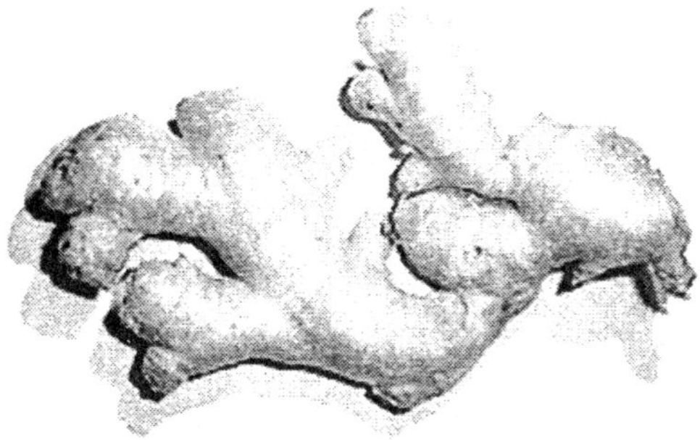

Ginger is grown throughout the tropical areas of the world. The most expensive and highest quality varieties generally come from Australia, South India, and Jamaica, while most mass market ginger is grown in China.

Medical research has shown that ginger root is an effective treatment for nausea caused by motion sickness, morning sickness or other illness. Ginger root also contains many antioxidants. Powdered dried ginger root is made into pills for medicinal use. Chinese women traditionally eat ginger root during pregnancy to combat morning sickness. Ginger ale and ginger beer have been recommended as "stomach settlers" for generations in countries where the beverages are made. Ginger water was commonly used to avoid heat cramps in the United States in the past.

The chacteristic odor and flavor of ginger root is caused by a mixture of shogaol and gingerols, volatile oils that compose about 1%-3% by weight of fresh ginger. The gingerols have analgesic, sedative, antipyretic, antibacterial, and GI tract motility effects.

Ginger reduces nausea. It is on the GRAS list from FDA.

Gastrointesinal; stimulates circulation; a useful diaphoretic, promoting perspiration. As a gargle it can give temporary relief of sore throats.

Ginkgo Leaf (Ginkgo Biloba)

Circulatory; brain circulation, anti-inflammatory, vasoddilatory, relaxant, has been suggested in the following conditions: vertigo, tinnitus, inner ear disturbances including partial deafness,impairment of memory and ability to concentrate, diminished intellectual capacity and alertness as a result of insufficient circulation, Raynaud's disease, arterial circulatory disturbances due to aging,

Ginseng, American Wild (Panax quinquefolia)

An adaptogen (helps the system adapt to a variety of changes); increases energy; decreases blood pressure. contraindicated during pregnancy.

Ginseng, Siberian (Eleutherococcus senticosus)

An adaptogen; lowers stress; both raises and/or lowers blood sugar43 as needed. contraindicated during pregnancy.

Ginsenosides

A class of triterpene saponins found in ginseng and other Panax species.

Glycogen

A polysaccharide, also called animal starch. The form in which carbohydrates are stored in the animal body.

Glycoprotein

A polysaccharide, also called animal starch. The form in which carbohydrates are stored in the animal body.

2. A compound consisting of a carbohydrate and a protein.

Glycosides

Glycosides, or sugar ethers, are a complex grouping which can be broken down to yield one or more sugars (glycones), plus a non-sugar component (aglycones). It is important to note that glycosides are not a major classification of phytochemicals, as are alkaloids, carbohydrates, phenols and terpenoids. However, it is often when a phytochemical is in its glycosidic form that a constituent may have a specific therapeutic action. Neucleotide glycosides, in combination with particular compounds, create specific glycosides in plants, the distinction between which is signified by a C-, S-, N-, or

O-. The letters indicate that the formation of the glycoside is dependent on interaction with Carbon, Sulphur, Nitrogen, or alcohol/phenol components, respectively (Evans, 281). Given this mutability, glycosides can occur in any of the major phytochemical classifications, because a sugar ether can bind itself to molecules in a myriad of ways.Glycosides are most commonly classified according to the chemical nature of the aglycone, and have vast medicinal applications as they are found in almost every therapeutic class.

Some phytochemical groups, such as anthraquinone phenols, normally do contain glycosides, so they are nicknamed anthraquinone glycosides. Alcohol glycosides have been used as antirheumatics and analgesics. Salicin, from Salix spp., is the glycosidic precursor to what is transformed to salicylic acid in our bodies. Salicylic acid is an anodyne: Ultimately, salicylic acid was synthesized to become today's aspirin.

Known primarily for their laxative actions, anthraquinone glycosides were found after the aglycones (a non-sugar component) of anthraquinones had been obtained upon hydrolysis. Both glycones and aglycones of anthracene derivation are polyphenols containing the red or purple pigment found in senna, cascara, rheum, and aloe, for example.

Flavonoid glycosides are yellow pigments in flowers and plants which have demonstrated antiinflammatory, anti-allergic effects, antithrombotic and vasoprotective properties. These plant constituents exert antioxidant effects on free radicals in the body. Related to flavonoid glycosides are the anthocyanidins and anthocyanins, mentioned under the phenol heading.

Lactone glycosides, a.k.a. Coumarin glycosides are very fragrant: they are the source, for instance, of freshly-mown hay scents (ibid.). Medicinally, coumarin glycosides have been shown to have hemorrhagic, antifungicidal, and antitumor activities. The lactone glycoside dicumarol is known as an anticoagulant.

Cardiac glycosides, come from triterpenoid groups and their action on the heart is still under investigation. It is known, however, that the cardiac glycosides do exert a specific action on the myocardial muscle and allay myocardial infarction.

Digitalis, from the foxglove plant, is an allopathic prescription. (Planta Medica, 1993, 539.)

Cyanogenic glycosides, which initially contain hydrogen cyanide (HCN) compounds, are toxic to unadapted farm animals and humans. However, some have been found to be of cytotoxic interest in cancer research. Originally, these glycosides were probably developed so that a plant could defend itself from herbivores. The cyanide content, referred to as a bound toxin, only occurs in some of the 1000 or so plants which initially produce cyanohydrin upon hydrolysis (Harborne and Baxter, 84). Detection of the presence of cyanide is accomplished through smell or by its yellow to brownish-red reaction with moist picrate paper. Prunasin, to illustrate, is a cyanogenic glycoside occurring in Wild Cherry Bark, a botanical which has been used since the late 1700's as a cough sedative and medicinal flavorant (Evans, 538). Diagnostic caution: if the amygdalin is present with benzaldehyde following hydrolysis, the agent is an aldehyde glycoside.

2. A plant constituent that on hydrolysis yields a sugar and one or more additional products; depending on the sugar liberated, glycosides are designated either galactosides or glucosides.

A hormone capable of promoting gonadal growth and function, such as stimulation of follicular growth.

3. Any of various kinds of molecules (including flavonoids) which have a sugar group attached to the main part of the molecule. The molecule without the sugar is known as the aglycone. A glycoside that has glucose as its sugar unit is called a glucoside.

GMP Critical Parameter

A parameter that has a direct effect on product quality.

GMP Facility

A production facility or clinical trial materials pilot plant for the manufacture of pharmaceutical products. It includes the manufacturing space, the storage warehouse for raw and finished product, and support lab areas. A GMP facility operates under the guidelines established by the CFR (Code of

Federal Regulations) Title 21, Parts 225 (Current Good Manufacturing for Medicated Feeds - Subpart B), and Part 226 (Current Good Manufacturing Practice for Type A Medicated Articles - Subpart B).

Gokhru

There are two types of Gokhru available from two different plants. The small Gokhru is the fruit obtained from *Tribulus terrestris* Linn.

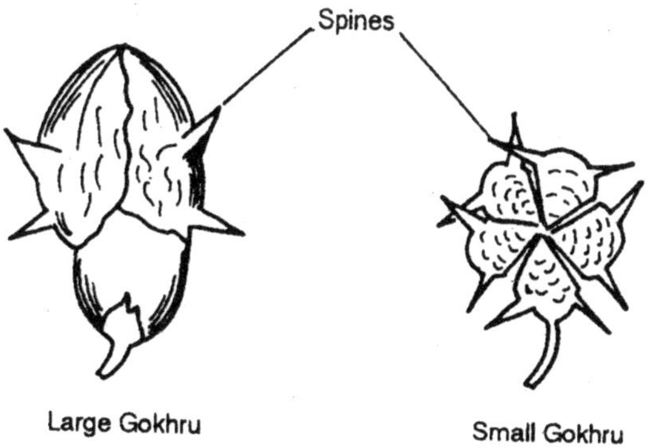

Large and Small Gokhru

Goldenseal (Hydrastis canadensis)

Antimicrobial; a bitter herb whose root is an anticarrhal; tonic; used as a antibiotic44; contains berberine effective against Helobacter pylori (often responsible for recurrent ulcers) and giardia; effective against gram-positive bacteria such as streptococcus and staph45, and gram-negative bacteria such as Escherichia coli46; treats eczema and ringworm (applied topically) reduces inflammation of the eyes47; contraindicated during pregnancy.

Golgi Bodies

Very small particles composed of membrane aggregates and responsible for the secretion of certain enzymes and macromolecules. Golgi bodies are the deposition and packaging site for many excreted products.

"Green Labeling"

Certification programs calling for voluntary compliance with established environmental standards in exchange for higher prices or greater market access, or both.

Good Engineering Practice (GEP)

A combination of standards, specifications, codes, regulatory and industrial guidelines as well as accepted engineering and design methods intended to design, construct, operate, and maintain pharmaceutical and/or biotechnology facilities taking into account not only regulatory compliance but also safety, economics, environmental protection and operability. Standards and specifications are provided by recognized sources such as established engineering and architectural contractors as well as pharmaceutical companies. Codes are provided by local, state, or federal jurisdictions and/or insurance companies. Guidelines are issued by professional societies, industrial organizations, or regulatory agencies. Engineering design methods have been established throughout the engineering educational system.

Good Large Scale Practice Organism (GLSP)

The National Institutes of Health (NIH) specifies physical containment levels and defines Biosafety Levels for Large Scale in their "Guidelines for Research Involving Recombinant DNA Molecules" - Appendix K - May 1999. Level of physical containment recommended for large-scale (more than 10 liters of culture) research or production involving viable, non-pathogenic, and non-toxigenic recombinant strains derived from host organisms that have an extended history of safe large scale use. Likewise, the GLSP level of physical containment is recommended for organisms that have a built-in environmental limitation that permits optimum growth in large-scale bioreactors, but limited survival if released to the environment.

Gram

One ounce contains 28.35 grams (g); a milligram (mg) is 1/1000 of a gram, so one ounce contains 28,349.5 milligrams. A microgram (µg) is 1/1,000,000 of a gram; one ounce contains 28,349,523 micrograms. Here's a great unit converter for translating one measurement into another.

H

Hairpin

A double helical region formed by base pairing between adjacent (inverted) complementary sequences in a single strand of RNA or DNA..

Half-life

The time it takes for half of a given quantity of a particular compound to decompose or transform into other compounds.

Haloenzyme

An enzyme that contains a non-protein component.

Halogen

One of the chlorine group (bromine, chlorine, fluorine, iodine) of elements, all univalent; they form monobasic acids with hydrogen, and their hydroxides (fluorine forms none) are monobasic acids. The radioactive element, astatine, also belongs to the halogen group.

Halophile

An organism that displays accelerated growth or is dependent on high salt concentrations.

Handshake

Requires the recipient of an electronic data record to acknowledge to the sender that the record has been received.

Handwritten Signature

The scripted name or legal mark of an individual handwritten by that individual and executed or adopted with the present intention to authenticate a writing in a permanent form. The act of signing with a writing or marking instrument such as a pen or stylus is preserved. The scripted name or legal mark, while conventionally applied to paper, may also be applied to other devices that capture the name or mark. (also see:

Haploid

A single set of chromosomes (half the full set of genetic material), present in the egg and sperm cells of animals and in the egg and pollen cells of plants. Human beings have 23 chromosomes in their reproductive cells.

Hardness

Concentration of calcium and magnesium salts in water. Hardness originally referred to the soap-consuming power of water; as such it is sometimes also taken to include iron and manganese. "Permanent hardness" also known as "noncarbonated hardness " is the excess of hardness over alkalinity. "Temporary hardness" also known as "carbonated hardness" is equal or less than the alkalinity. Permanent hardness can cause boiler or pipe scale and failure of reverse osmosis membranes.

Harvesting

The separation of cells from growth media. It can be accomplished by filtration, precipitation, or centrifugation.

Hazardous Chemical Reaction

A reaction which generates pressure or byproducts which could cause injury, illness or harm to humans, domestic animals, livestock or wildlife.

Hazardous Occupancy - Group H - (California Building Code) Group H occupancies include buildings or structures, or portions thereof, that involve the manufacturing, processing, generation or storage of materials that constitute a high fire, explosion, or health hazard. There are eight divisions in this Group:

1. Division 1 - Occupancies with a quantity of material in the building exceeding regulation set limits and that present a high explosion hazard, such as blasting agents, fireworks, black powder, certain oxidizers and detonatable unstable (reactive) materials, and other materials (refer to Code for more details).
2. Division 2 - Occupancies where combustible dust is manufactured, used, or generated in such a manner that concentrations and conditions creates fire or explosion potential, or occupancies where materials exceeding regulation set limits present a moderate explosion hazard or a hazard from accelerated burning, such as some organic peroxides, pyrophoric gases, flammable or oxidizing gases, some nondetonatable unstable (reactive) materials, and other materials (refer to Code for more details).
3. Division 3 - Occupancies where flammable solids, other than combustible dust, are manufactured, used or generated, or occupancies where materials exceeding regulation set limits present a high physical hazard, such as some organic peroxides and oxidizers, pyrophoric liquids or solids, flammable solids in storage, flammable or oxidizing cryogenic fluids, and other materials.
4. Division 4 - Repair garages not classified as Group S, Division 3 Occupancies.
5. Division 5 - Aircraft repair hangars not classified as Group S, Division 5 Occupancies, and heliports.
6. Division 6 - Semiconductor fabrication facilities and comparable research and development areas in which hazardous production materials (HPM) are used and the aggregate quantity of materials exceeds those set by regulations. Such facilities and areas shall be designed and constructed following a different set of regulations.
7. Division 7 - Occupancies having quantities of materials in excess of those set by regulations, and that are health hazards, such as corrosives (except stationary lead-acid battery systems), toxic and highly toxic materials, irritants, sensitizers, and other health hazards.
8. Division 8 - Laboratories and similar areas used for scientific experimentation or research having quantities of materials not in excess of those set by regulations, and not otherwise classified as Group B, Division 2 Occupancies.

Hazardous Substance

A substance which by reason of being explosive, flammable, toxic, poisonous, corrosive, oxidizing, irritant or otherwise harmful, is likely to cause injury.

Haze

The abnormal appearance of a localized diminishing in brightness or luster of a surface when compared to the adjacent surfaces.

Health Hazard

Classification of a chemical for which there is statistically significant evidence based on at least one study conducted in accordance with established scientific principles that acute or chronic health effects may occur in exposed persons. The term "health hazard" includes chemicals that are carcinogens, toxic or highly toxic agents, reproductive toxins, irritants, corrosives, sensitizers, hepatotoxins, nephrotoxins, neurotoxins, agents that act on the hematopoietic system, and agents that damage the lungs, skin, eyes or mucous membranes.

Heat

A form of energy associated with the motion of atoms or molecules in solids and capable of being transmitted through solid and fluid media by conduction, through fluid media by convection, and through empty space by radiation. Two important characteristics of heat are:

1. Heat cannot be destroyed, only transferred from on body to another, or converted to another form of energy.
2. Heat always flows from the warmer to the colder substance.

Heat Affected Zone (HAZ)

That portion of the base metal that has not been melted but whose microstructure or mechanical properties have been altered by the heat of welding, brazing, soldering, forming, or cutting.

Heat Labile

Able to be destroyed or altered by high temperature. Heat labile pharmaceuticals are sterilized by filtration.

Heat Number

An alphanumeric identification of a stated tonnage of metal obtained from a continuous melting in a foundry furnace.

Heat of Vaporization

The amount of heat needed to change a unit volume from a liquid to a vapor at a given pressure without a temperature change.

Heavy Metals

High molecular weight metal ions, such as lead. Known for their interference with many processes, and "poisoning" of catalysts, membranes, and resins.

HeLa Cells

An established line of human cervical carcinoma cells used to study the biochemistry and genetics of human cell growth.

Helix

A spiral, staircase-like, structure with a repeating pattern described by two simultaneous operations, rotation, and translation. It is the natural conformation of many biological polymers.

Hematin

An iron protoporphyrin differing from heme in that the central iron atom is in the ferric (Fe+++) rather than the ferrous (Fe++) state; the prosthetic group of methemoglobin.

Hemodynamic

Referring to the circulatory system.

Hemoglobin

The red, respiratory conjugated protein of erythrocytes, consisting of approximately 6 percent heme and 94 percent globin (a protein).

Hemophilia

A hereditary, plasma-coagulation disorder, principally

affecting males but transmitted by females, and characterized by excessive, sometimes spontaneous, bleeding.

Hemopoietic

Pertaining to or related to the formation of blood cells.

HEPA (High Efficiency Particulate Air) Filters

Filters with a minimum efficiency of 99.97% for 0.3μm particle size as determined by test. The test can be by the monodispersed dioctyl phthalate (DOP) method or other equally sensitive method. When operated at design velocity, larger and smaller particles are captured at higher efficiencies. HEPA filters are made of compressed and bonded micro-fiberglass or Teflon® corrugated to produce a high surface area in a small area panel of filter medium. Employed in unidirectional airflow benches, air handlers, and as terminal air supply filters in cleanrooms.

Heparin

A sulphur containing polysaccharide that stops blood from clotting by preventing the conversion of prothrombin to thrombin and by neutralizing thrombin. It is contained in the mast cells and is extractable from various tissues, notably the lung.

Hepatotoxin

A toxin that is destructive to parenchymal (specific tissue) cells of the liver.

Heredity

Transfer of genetic information from parent cells to progeny.

Heterotrophs

One of two categories in which microorganisms are classified on the basis of their carbon source. Heterotrophs use organic compounds such as carbohydrates, lipids, and hydrocarbons as a carbon and energy source.

Heterozygosity

The presence of different alleles at one or more loci on homologous chromosomes.

High Purity Process Systems

The equipment that includes the stainless steel vessels, tube, pipe, fittings, and valves used to manufacture and transport drug products.

Histamine

A substance produced from the amino acid histidine, which occurs in the body; functions include increasing gastric secretion, dilation of capillaries, and contraction of bronchial smooth muscle.

HMG CoA reductase

3-hydroxy-3-methylglutaryl-conenzyme A reductase, a microsomal enzyme that is a rate-limiting step in cholesterol biosynthesis. HMG-CoA reductase is a prime target for pharmacological intervention.

Hold-up Volume

The volume of liquid remaining in a vessel or piping system after it has been allowed to drain.

Hollow Fiber

Refers to reverse osmosis and ultrafiltration membranes formed into small diameter (about 0.05" I.D.) tubes. The inner surface is a very thin (RO or UF) membrane skin supported by a thicker porous outer layer that gives the tube its strength. Hollow fibers are used in bundles of 1,000 or more in a single cartridge shell. Water is forced through the center (upstream surface) of each tube and purified permeate is collected from the outer wall (downstream surface).

Homeobox

A short stretch of nucleotides whose base sequence is virtually identical in all the genes that contains it. It has been found in many organisms from fruit flies to human beings. In the fruit fly, a homeobox appears to determine when particular groups of genes are expressed during development.

Homeopathy

School of medicine founded by Dr. Samuel Christian Friederich

Hahnemann, based on the theory that large doses of drugs that cause symptoms of a disease will cure the symptoms when administered in small doses. Loosely based on the notion that "like cures like."

Homologous Chromosome

Chromosome containing the same linear gene sequences as another, each derived from one parent.

Homology

Similarity in DNA or protein sequences between individuals of the same species or among different species.

Honeysuckle Flowers (Lonicera periclymenum)

Laxative; expectorant.

Horehound (Marrubium vulgare)

A cough remedy48; used to facilitate healing of bronchitis and asthma; expels mucous from the lungs and throat.

Hormone

A substance that originates in an organ, gland, or part that is conveyed through the circulation to another part of another hormone.

2. A type of chemical messenger, occurring both in plants and animals, that acts to inhibit or excite metabolic activities. Its site of production is distant from the site of biological activity.

Horseradish

Horseradish *(Armoracia rusticana, syn. Cochlearia armoracia)* is a perennial plant of the Brassicaceae family, which includes mustard and cabbages. The plant is probably native to southeastern Europe and western Asia, but is popular around the world today. It grows up to 1.5 metres (five feet) tall and is mainly cultivated for its large white, tapering root, although the leaves are also edible.

Its root is used as a vegetable or condiment, and has at times been used as the bitter herbs in the Passover meal in some Jewish communities. Horseradish, sometimes blended with cream, is often served with roast or boiled beef or sausages, as well as smoked fish. Horseradish is also used in some prepared mustards. Also, much of what is styled wasabi is actually common horseradish dyed green.

The horseradish root itself has hardly any aroma. When cut or grated, however, enzymes from the damaged plant cells break down sinigrin (a glucosilinate) to produce allylisothiocyanate (mustard oil), which irritates the sinuses and eyes. Once grated, use horseradish immediately or mix it in vinegar, as the root darkens and loses its pungency and becomes unpleasantly bitter when exposed to air and heat.

Over two thirds of the world's horseradish is said to be grown in a small region around Collinsville, Illinois in the US, the self-styled "Horseradish Capital of the World", whence it is even exported overseas as a gourmet version of the product to places more renowned for consumption of the root.

It has been speculated that the word is a partial translation of its German name Meerrettich. The element Meer (meaning 'ocean, sea') is pronounced like the English word mare, which might have been reinterpreted as horseradish. On the other hand, many English plant names have "horse" as an element denoting strong or coarse, so the etymology of the English word (which is attested in print from at least 1597) is uncertain.

Horseradish contains potassium, calcium, magnesium and phosporus, as well as volatile oils, such as mustard oil, which is antibiotic. Fresh, the plant contains 177,9 mg/100 g of vitamin C. The enzyme horseradish peroxidase, found in the plant, is used extensively in molecular biology in antibody amplification and detection, among other things.

Horseradish was cultivated in antiquity. Cato discusses the plant in his treatises on agriculture, and a mural in Pompeii showing the plant has survived until today. It is probably the plant mentioned by Pliny under the name of Amoracia, and recommended by him for its medicinal qualities, and possibly the Wild Radish, or raphanos agrios of the Greeks.

Both root and leaves were universally used as a medicine during the Middle Ages, and as a condiment in Denmark and Germany. William Turner mentions horseradish as Red Cole in his "Herbal" (1551-1568), but not as a condiment. In "The Herball, or Generall Historie of Plantes" (1597), John Gerard describes it under the name of raphanus rusticanus, stating that it occurs wild in several parts of England. After referring to its medicinal uses, he says: the Horse Radish stamped with a little vinegar put thereto, is commonly used among the Germans for sauce to eate fish with and such like meates as we do mustarde. Before pepper and chiles became widely available, horseradish and mustard were the only sharp spices known in Europe.

Host

An organism in which another organism spends part or all of its life cycle.

Host Vector (HV) System

The host is the organism into which a gene from another organism is transplanted. The guest gene is carried by a vector, which is a larger DNA molecule, such as a plasmid, or a virus into which that gene is genetically engineered and which then propagates in the host. NIH Guidelines under Appendix E. - Certified Host-Vector Systems contains a list of derivatives host-vector systems previously classified as Host-Vector 1 Systems or Host-Vector 2 Systems, they are: Bacillus subtilis, Saccharomyces Cerevisiae, Escherichia coli, Neurospora crassa, Streptomyces, and Pseudonomas putida.

HPLC

High Pressure or High Performance Liquid Chromatography. Liquid chromatography employing high pressure and short columns to effect separation of constituents of a mixture.

2. Sometimes called high-performance liquid chromatography, is a separation technique based on a solid stationary phase and a liquid mobile phase. Separations (into distinct bands) are achieved by partition, adsorption, or ion-exchange processes, depending upon the type of stationary phase used. Each band is then profiled as the solvent flows through a UV detector, or by fluorescence, or refractive index detectors.

HSA (Human Serum Albumin)

The main protein constituent of human serum. It has no prosthetic group and is soluble in water and dilute salt solution. It is sometimes used in the treatment of shock, hypoproteinemia, and erythroblastosis fetalis.

Human Gene Therapy

Insertion of normal DNA directly into cells to correct a genetic defect.

Human Genome

The full collection of genes needed to produce a human being.

Human Genome Initiative

Collective name for several projects begun in 1986 by DOE to:
1. Create an ordered set of DNA segments from known chromosomal locations.
2. Develop new computational methods for analyzing genetic map and DNA sequence.
3. Develop new techniques and instruments for detecting and analyzing DNA.

This DOE initiative is now known as the Human Genome Program. The national effort, led by DOE and NIH, is known as the Human Genome Project.

Huntington's Disease

An adult-onset disease characterized by progressive mental and physical deterioration; it is caused by an inherited dominant gene mutation.

Hyaluronic acid

Acid mucopolysaccharide found in the ground substance of connective tissue that acts as a binding and protective agent. Also found in synovial fluid, and vitreous and aqueous tumors.

Hyaluronidase

An enzyme that catalyses the hydrolysis of hyaluronic acid, which increases the permeability of connective tissue by dissolving the substances that hold body cells together.

Hybrid Systems

Combination of electronic and paper records, common in today's analytical labs, in which raw data is recorded electronically to reconstruct the analysis, but the final results are printed and signed on paper. FDA does not prohibit hybrid systems but has expressed some concerns about their usefulness.

Hybridization

The process of joining two complementary strands of DNA or one each of DNA and RNA to form a double-stranded molecule.

Hybridoma

A hybrid cell resulting from the fusion of a specific antibody producing spleen cell with a myeloma cell. The hybrid cell has the growth characteristics of the myeloma component and the antibody secreting characteristics of the spleen cell and will multiply to become a source of large quantities of pure, monoclonal antibody.

Hydrogen Peroxide (H_2O_2)

A colorless, heavy, strongly oxidizing, unstable liquid used principally in aqueous solutions as an antiseptic, bleaching agent, oxidizing agent, and laboratory reagent. In the vapor phase, as an airborne sterilant.

Hydrogen bond

A relatively weak kind of chemical bond where there is an attraction between a hydrogen atom on one molecule and an oxygen or nitrogen atom on another. Helps to stabilize the shape of molecules such as proteins (including enzymes) and DNA; accounts for the 'surface tension' of water.

Hydrolysis

A chemical reaction between water and organic compounds, particularly esters, ketones, and alcohols. This reaction can lead to breakdown of some proteins.

Hydroxyl group

A hydroxyl group is a functional group consisting of an oxygen atom bonded to a hydrogen atom (-OH). It is very common in biomolecules.

Hydrophilic

Having a strong affinity for water. Its opposite, hydrophobic.

Hydrophobic

Non-wetting; water repelling.

Hydrotest

A pressure test of piping, pressure vessels, or pressure-containing parts, usually performed by pressurizing the internal volume with water at a pressure determined by the applicable code or to test the integrity of a process system.

Hygienic

Of, or pertaining to, equipment and piping systems that by design, materials of construction, and operation provide for the maintenance of cleanliness (pyrogen free but not sterile) so that products produced by these systems will not adversely affect human or animal health.

Hygienic Clamp Joint

A tube outside diameter union consisting of two neutered ferrules having flat faces with a concentric groove and mating gasket that is secured with a clamp, providing a nonprotruding, recessless product contact surface. Tri-clamp™ is a Tri-Clover proprietary name; consequently, it should not be used to describe the above-mentioned fitting unless that particular brand is used.

Hygroscopicity

The affinity for absorbing water.

Hypochlorite

A weak, unstable salt of hypochlorous acid used in aqueous solutions as a bleach, oxidizer, deodorant, and disinfectant.
Immune Response
The production of antibodies (humoral response) or particular types of cytotoxic lymphoid cells (cell-mediated response) on challenge with an antigen.

Hyoscymus

Hyoscymus is the dried leaves and flowering tops of *Hyoscymus niger* containing not less than 0.05 percent of th alkaloids of hyoscymus calculated as hyoscyamine.

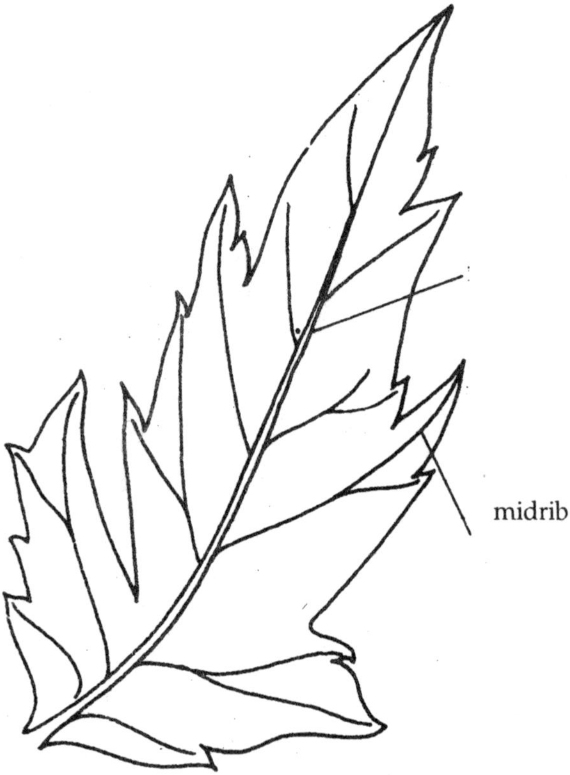

Hyoscymus

Hyperkalemia

Excess potassium in the blood.

Hyperlipidemia

Increase of lipids in the blood.

Hypothalamus

Deep brain structure whose secretions are important for the regulation of metabolic activities and the discharge of inhibiting and releasing hormones.

I

Immunocompromised

Having an immune system incapable of responding to pathogens or tissue damage.

Immuno Electrophoresis

The separation of different antigen-antibody systems by diffusion in an agar gel; a separate precipitation band in the gel detects each system.

Immunotimulant

A substance or agent that causes antibody formation.

Immunity

The state of an organism in which protection from many infectious diseases is afforded by prior exposure to the infectious agents.

Immunogen

A substance that is capable of causing antibody formation.

Immunoglobulin (Ig)

A member of a class of proteins that functions as an antibody. The wide range of different specifities of antibodies depends on subtle differences in their structure.

Immunoglobulin A (IgA)

The body's first line of defense against infectious diseases and is present in seromucous secretions such as saliva, tears, nasal fluids, sweat and secretions of the lung and genito-urinary and gastro-intestinal tracts.

Immunoglobulin (IgA, IgD, IgE, IgG, and IgM)

A class of serum proteins rich in antibodies. Often used, along with the more specific monoclonal antibodies, in diagnostic reagents in the health field.

Immunology

The study of how the body defends itself against disease.

Immunoproteins

All the proteins concerned with the immune system (antibodies, interferon, and cytokines).

Imprinting

A biochemical phenomenon that determines, for certain genes, which one of the pair of alleles, the mother's or the father's, will be active in that individual.

Impurity

Any component present in the intermediate or API (Active Pharmaceutical Ingredient) that is not the desired entity. It may be either process or product related.

Impurity Profile

A description of the identified and unidentified impurities present in a typical batch of API (Active Pharmaceutical Ingredient) produced by a specific controlled production process. It includes the identity or some qualitative analytical designation (e.g. retention time), the range of each impurity observed, and type of each identified impurity. For each API there should be an impurity profile describing the identified and unidentified impurities present in a typical batch. The impurity profile is normally dependent upon the process or origin of the API.

Inactive Ingredient

Any component other than an active ingredient.

Inactivation

Any process that destroys the ability of a specific microbiological agent or eukaryotic cell to self-replicate.

Incidental Release

The discharge of a microbilogical agent or eukaryotic cell from a containment system that is expected when the system is appropriately designed and properly operated and maintained. Incidental releases are de minimis in nature.

Inclusion Body

Condensed particles of protein formed inside E. coli and other bacteria formed when the cells are forced to make large amounts of a product protein. The cells must be broken to harvest inclusion bodies.

Inclusions

Particles of foreign material in a metallic matrix. The particles are usually compounds such as oxides, sulfides, or silicates, but may be any substance foreign to and essentially insoluble in the matrix.

IND (Investigational New Drug) Application

A document filed with the FDA prior to clinical trial of a new drug. It gives a full description of the new drug, where and how is manufactured, all QC information, etc. The IND is followed by NDA (New Drug Application).

Indirect Impact System

An engineering system considered having no direct impact on product quality.

Inert

Does not dissolve in water or react chemically with other substances.

Infarct

A necrotic area of tissue resulting from failure of local blood supply.

Infected

Contaminated with extraneous biological agents and therefore capable of spreading infection.

Infectious

Capable of spreading from individual to individual by a variety of routes.

Infectious Agent

A biological organism that can establish a process of infection.

Infiltration

The entry of air from an adjoining room or from outdoors through wall and ceiling openings due to a difference in air pressure between the two areas.

Inflorescence

Inflorescence is a bunch of flower. Axis of flower is called peduncle depending upon the type of branch. It may be a different types such as mustard, spike (vasaka), umbel (coriander, cumin, fennel) and capitulum. Compositae is the largest family of flowering plants characterised by a capitulum inflorescence in which a large number of flowers are grouped in single head e.g. pyrethrum.

Informatics

The study of the application of computer and statistical techniques to the management of information. In genome projects, informatics includes the development of methods to search databases quickly, to analyze DNA sequence information, and to predict protein sequence and structure from DNA sequence data.

Infusion

The introduction of parenterals into a vein (intravenous).

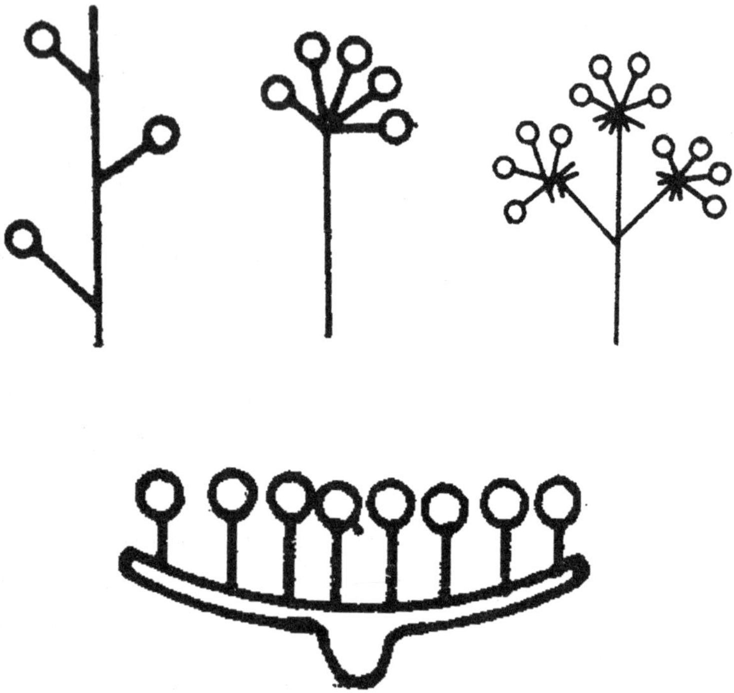

Inflorescence Types

In vitro

An experimental test or procedure conducted using isolated tissues, organs, cells, or cell preparations.

In vivo

An experimental test or procedure conducted using whole live organisms.

Indole alkaloids

A class of alkaloids (see), which incorporate indole (2,3-benzopyrrole) into its structure.

Injection

A preparation intended for parenteral administration and/or

constituting or diluting a parenteral article prior to administration. The introduction of parenterals may be into the subcutaneous cellular tissue (subcutaneous or hypodermic), or the muscular tissue (Intramuscular).

In-Line

An integral part of the flow path. In a fluid stream, something is said to be in-line if the entire fluid stream flows directly through or past it.

In-Process Control

Checks performed during production in order to monitor and if necessary to adjust the process and/or to ensure that the intermediate or API (Active Pharmaceutical Ingredient) conforms to its specification. (also called Process Control)

Innocuous

Safe, not contaminated.

Inoculum

1. Fermentation: an aliquot of a pure culture of microorganism added to the primary seed tank to initiate fermentation.

In vitro

Literally, 'in glass': generally refers to scientific studies performed on cells cultured in Petri dishes. The results of in vitro studies suggest, but cannot predict, the effects a substance will have on a living organisms (such as a mouse or human being). This is contrasted to in vivo, which means 'in the living organism.'

Isomer

Two compounds are isomers of each other when they have the same number and kinds of atoms, but those atoms are arranged in different ways.

Ipecacuanha

Ipecacuanha consists of the dried, enlarged adventitious roots of *Cephaelis ipecacuanha* (Brot.) A Rich.

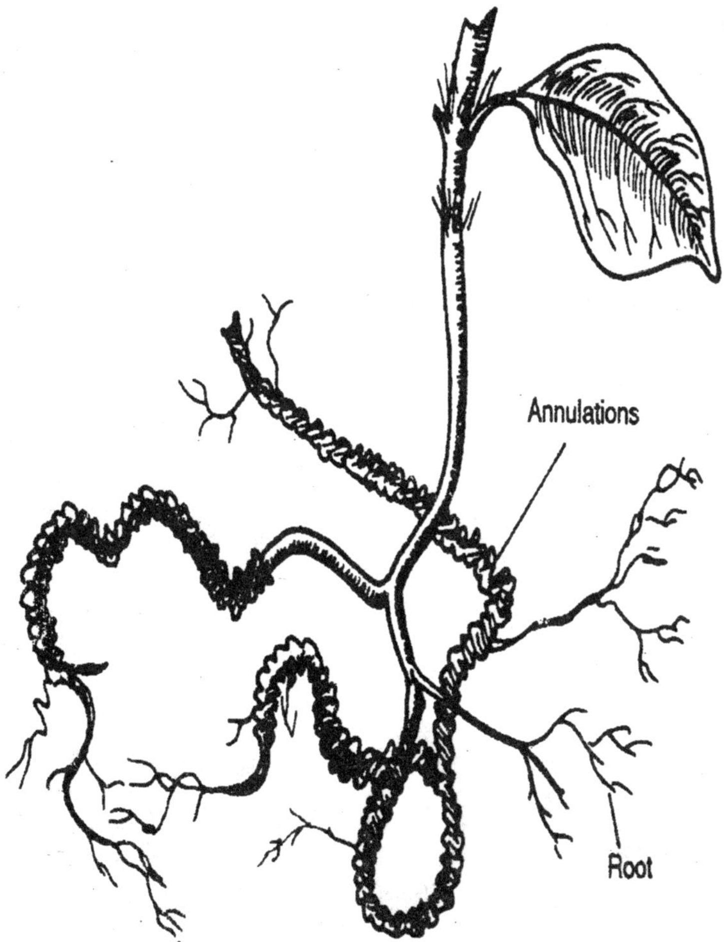

Ipecacuanha Root

Ispaghula

The drug consists of seeds of *Plantago ovata Forsk.*

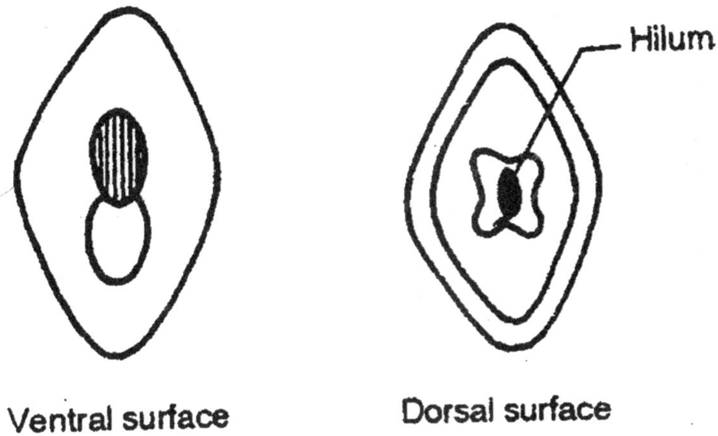

Ispaghula

J

Juniper

Junipers are coniferous plants in the genus Juniperus of the cypress family Cupressaceae. There are about 50-55 species of juniper, widely distributed throughout the northern hemisphere, from the arctic, south to tropical Africa in the Old World, and to the mountains of Central America in the New World.

Junipers vary in size and shape from tall trees to 20-40 m tall, to columnar or low spreading shrubs with long trailing branches. They are evergreen with either needle-like and/or scale-like leaves. They can be either monoecious or dioecious. The female seed cones are very distinctive, with fleshy, fruit-like coalescing scales which fuse together to form a "berry"-like structure, 4-27 mm long, with 1-12 unwinged, hard-shelled seeds. In some species these "berries" are red-brown or orange but in most they are blue; they are often aromatic (for their use as a spice, see Juniperus communis). The seed maturation time varies between species from 6-18 months after pollination. The male cones are similar to those of other Cupressaceae, with 6-20 scales; most shed their pollen in early spring, but some species pollinate in the autumn.

Many junipers (e.g. J. chinensis, J. virginiana) have two types of leaves: seedlings and some twigs of older trees have needle-like leaves 5-25 mm long; and the leaves on mature plants are (mostly) tiny (2-4 mm long), overlapping and scale-like. When juvenile foliage occurs on mature plants, it is most often found on shaded shoots, with adult foliage in full sunlight. Leaves on fast-growing 'whip' shoots are often intermediate between juvenile and adult.

In some species (e.g. J. communis, J. squamata), all the foliage is of the juvenile needle-like type, with no scale leaves. In some of these (e.g. J. communis), the needles are jointed at the base, in others (e.g. J. squamata), the needles merge smoothly with the stem, not being jointed.

The needle-leaves of junipers are hard and sharp, making the juvenile foliage very prickly to handle. This can be a valuable identification feature in seedlings, as the otherwise very similar juvenile foliage of cypresses (Cupressus, Chamaecyparis) and other related genera is soft and not prickly.

K

Karyotype

A photomicrograph of an individual's chromosomes arranged in a standard format showing the number, size, and shape of each chromosome type. It is used in low-resolution physical mapping to correlate gross chromosomal abnormalities with the characteristics of specific diseases.

Keratins

Insoluble protective or structural proteins consisting of parallel polypeptide chains in a-helical or b-conformation.

Ketose

A simple monosaccharide having its carbonyl groups at other than a terminal position. Kilobase (kb) Unit of length for DNA fragments equal to 1000 nucleotides (kilo base pairs of DNA).

Kinase

An enzyme catalyzing phosphorylation of an acceptor molecule by adenosine triphosphate (ATP).

L

LD50

Median lethal dose of a substance, the amount that will kill 50% of the animals receiving the dose.

Labile

Unstable or unsteady; not fixed; characterized by adaptability to alteration or modification, i.e., relatively easily changed, as in cleavage of a molecule or molecular rearrangement in a compound or complex chemical material.

LAL (Limulus Amoebocyte Lysate)

A material obtained by rupturing the cellular components of the blood of a horseshoe crab (Limulus Poliphemus). This material coagulates in the presence of LPS (lypopolysaccharides) and is a test used to quantitate bacterial endotoxins (pyrogens).

Laminar Airflow

(also see: Unidirectional Airflow)

Laminar Airflow - Clean Work Station

A workstation in which the unidirectional airflow characteristics predominate throughout the entire airspace with a minimum of eddies (turbulence) to jeopardize critical surfaces.

Laminar Flow

Non-turbulent fluid flow is usually considered laminar if the Reynolds number is less than 2000 in a pipe. Depending upon many possible varying conditions, the flow may be laminar at a Reynolds number as low as 1,200 or as high as 40,000; however, such conditions are not experienced in normal practice. In the pharmaceutical industry, this term incorrectly refers to the air discharge of a clean air bench or wall.

LAN (Local Area Network)

Networks with computers geographically close together (that is, in the same building).

Langelier Index

A measure of the degree of saturation of calcium carbonate in water that is based on pH, alkalinity and hardness. If the Langelier Index is negative, the water is corrosive (pH value below 7 or acidic). If the Langelier Index is positive, calcium carbonate can precipitate out of solution to form scale (pH value above 7 or basic). The Langelier Index will vary for cold water and for warm water.

Latent Heat

The amount of heat needed to change a unit of substance, such as water, from a solid to a liquid without change in temperature or pressure.

Lay

In metallurgy, the direction of the predominant surface pattern ordinarily determined by the production method used.

Leach

To dissolve by the action of a moving liquid. For example, high purity water leaches trace impurities from glass vessels.

Lectin

One of several plant proteins that stimulate lymphocytes to proliferate.

Legacy Systems

Hardware and software applications in which a company has already invested considerable time and money. Legacy systems typically perform critical operations in companies for many years even though they may no longer use state-of-the-art technology. Replacing legacy systems can be disruptive and therefore requires careful planning and appropriate migration support from the manufacturer.

Lemon balm

Lemon Balm (Melissa officinalis), also known as Bee Balm, is a perennial herb from the mint family Lamiaceae, grown originally in Southern Europe. Its flavors come from the terpenes citronellal, citronellol, citral, and geraniol.

Its leaves have a gentle lemon scent, related to mint. At the end of the summer, little white flowers full of nectar appear. These attracts bees, hence the name "Melissa" (Greek for 'bee'). The stems of the plant die off at the start of the winter, but shoot up again in spring.

Leptospira

A genus of the family Treponemataceae, thin coiled organisms, flagellated at the extremities, one or both of which are bent back like a hook. Both pathogenic and innocent forms have been isolated.

Leukemia

Cancer that begins in developing blood cells in the bone marrow.

Leukocyte

A general name for white, nucleated blood cells found in the blood and lymphatic tissue.

2. White blood corpuscle; there are types, granulocytes, which include eosinophils and neutrophils, and agranulocytes, which include monocytes and lymphocytes.

Level of Product Protection

The level of protection required for an area based on an assessment by the manufacturer of contamination risk.

Licorice root (Glycyrrhiza glabra)

Soothes and heals mucous membranes in the intestinal tract49; treats ulcers50.

Ligand

A molecule or ion that is bound to protein.

A (usually smaller) molecule which binds to a (usually larger) molecule such as an enzyme or protein, and is either transformed into something else or initiates a metabolic process (i.e., a phytoestrogen - the ligand - binds to an estrogen receptor - the protein - and initiates a process such as transcription of a particular gene).

Ligase

An enzyme used to catalyze the joining of single-stranded DNA segments.

Linden Flowers (Tilia europaea)

A nervine, anti-spasmodic, anti-inflammatory, emmenagogue, hypotensive, diaphoretic, diuretic, astringent. Linden is well known as a relaxing remedy and in the treatment of raised blood pressure associated with nervous tension.

Linkage

The proximity of two or more markers (e.g., genes, RFLP markers) on a chromosome; the closer together the markers are, the lower the probability that they will be separated during DNA repair or replication processes (binary fission in prokaryotes, mitosis or meiosis in eukaryotes), and hence the greater the probability that they will be inherited together.

Linkage Map

A map of the relative positions of genetic loci on a chromosome, determined on the basis of how often the loci are inherited together. Distance is measured in centimorgans (cM).

Linseed

Linseed is the dried ripe seed of *Linum usitatissimum* Linn. belonging to family Linaceae.

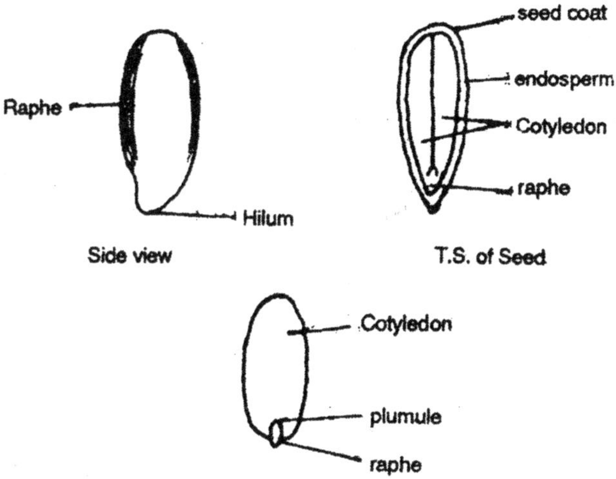

Linseed

Lipids

Fixed oils, fats, waxes, phosphatides, and lecithins, as members of the lipid group, are made up of esters of long-chain fatty

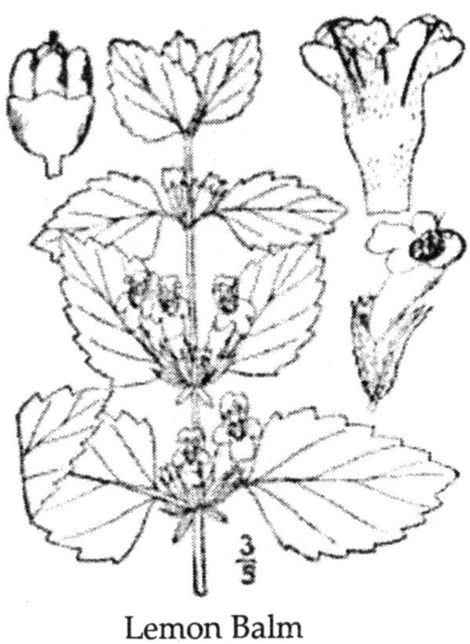

Lemon Balm

acids and alcohols which contain carbon, hydrogen, and oxygen. Fixed oils are liquid at normal temperature, fats are solid; however this distinction does not always come through, especially with differences in climate.

Lipids are often a main constituent in drugs, separated by expression from the crude vegetable (plant) matter and presented as drugs in the refined state. Plant seeds are the largest source (e.g. sesame seeds,almonds, linseed) of lipids. It is used as a flavouring in tisane and ice cream. It is also often paired with fruit dishes or candies.

This herb can be easy to cultivate in USDA Plant Hardiness Zones 4 through 8. In Zone 7 it can be harvested at least until the end of November.

Fatty or oily substance, insoluble in water. Includes fatty acids and triglycerides.

Lipid peroxidation

Oxidation of a lipid to a lipid peroxide; lipid peroxidation can damage membrane lipids of cells and tissues, and in fatty foods, can cause rancidity.

Hydrophobic biological compounds (fats and fatlike materials) that are insoluble in water, but soluble in nonpolar solvents such as benzene, chloroform, and ether. The major components in most lipids are fatty acids.

2. Lipids (such as the phospholipids in cell membranes and fatty acids in the bloodstream) are subject to attack by free radicals, which damage them by oxidation; this process is called lipid peroxidation. Lipid peroxidation has been implicated in atherosclerosis and other diseases. Antioxidants help protect against lipid peroxidation.

Lipophilic

Having an affinity for fat; in chemistry, fat-soluble.

Lipoprotein

Conjugated proteins consisting of simple proteins combined with lipid components such as cholesterol, phospholipids, or triglycerides. Classed as very low density (VLDL), low density (LDL), and high density (HDL).

2. A conjugated protein containing a lipid, prosthetic group.

Lipoprotein, high density (HDL)

Plasma lipids bound to albumin. Contains more protein than either very low density lipoprotein (VLDL) or low density lipoproteins (LDL).

Liposome

An artificial phospholipid vesicle. Liposomes can be useful for the enclosure of macromolecules such as nucleic acids or, after loading with an appropriate drug. They may be used therapeutically to achieve slow release of the drug into circulation.

Lipotropic factors

Compounds that promote the transportation and utilisation of fats and help to prevent accumulation of fats in the liver.

Liquorice

Liquorice (Br.) or licorice (Am.) is the plant, Glycyrrhiza glabra, in the Family Fabaceae from which a sweet flavour can be extracted. The liquorice plant is a legume related to beans and peas and native to southern Europe and parts of Asia. Very little commercial liquorice is grown in North America, but wild liquorice (G. lepidota) is quite common.

Liquorice is a highly effective cough remedy (expectorant), and has been used for this purpose since ancient times.

Liquorice extract is produced by boiling liquorice root and subsequently evaporating all or most of the water. Liquorice extract is traded both in solid and syrup form. Its active principle is glycyrrhizin, a sweetener more than 50 times as sweet as sucrose which also has active medical effects.

The flavour is common in medicines to disguise unpleasant flavours. Liquorice can also be found in many candies. The most popular in the United Kingdom and North America are very sweet Liquorice Allsorts. In continental Europe, however, far stronger, saltier, candies are preferred. It is well regarded as a low fat sweet. Liquorice is also found in some soft drinks.

Liquorice is a mild laxative. Also, the glycyrrhizin that it contains can lead to an increased blood pressure when liquorice candies are consumed in larger quantities (over 50 g per day).

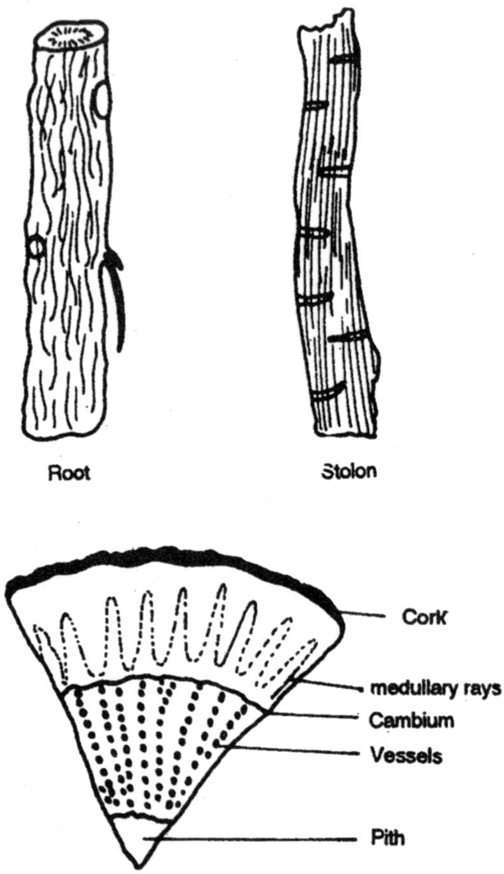

Liquorice

Localize

Determination of the original position (locus) of a gene or other marker on a chromosome.

Locus (pl. loci) The position on a chromosome of a gene or other chromosome marker; also, the DNA at that position. The use of locus is sometimes restricted to mean regions of DNA that are expressed.

Lomatium (Lomatium dissectum)

Antimicrobial.

Long-Range Restriction Mapping

Restriction enzymes are proteins that cut DNA at precise locations. Restriction maps depict the positions on chromosomes of restriction enzyme cutting sites. These are used as biochemical "signposts", or markers of specific areas along the chromosomes. The map will detail the positions on the DNA molecule that are cut by particular restriction enzymes.

Lower Flammability Level (LFL)

The minimum concentration of vapor in air at which propagation of flame will occur in the presence of an ignition source. LFL is sometimes referred to as LEL or Lower Explosive Limit.

LPS (Lipopolysaccharide)

Molecule found in the outer cell walls of some bacteria that trigger the immune response resulting in fever. Also referred to as pyrogens or as endotoxins, though, strictly speaking, they are not endotoxins but predominant components of endotoxins produced by gram-negative bacteria. Common cause of pyrogenic reactions in parenteral products.

Luteinizing hormone (LH)

Hormone secreted by anterior lobe of the pituitary that stimulates development of the corpus luteum.

Lymph

An alkaline fluid found in the lymphatic vessels and the cisterna chyli. It differs from blood in that red blood corpuscles are absent and the protein content is lower.

Lymphocyte

Cell present in the blood and lymphatic tissue, derived from the stem cells from which blood cells arise. They are the main source of providing the body with immune capabilities, by

means of humoral immunity produced by B cells and cell-mediated immunity produced by T cells.
2. A type of white blood cell accounting for 20-25% of the white cells in humans. They are mostly non-phagocytic and actively mobile and are continuously made in the bone marrow. They are the immediate precursors of all antibody-forming cells.

Lyophilization

Also known as freeze drying, it is a means of stabilizing wet substances by freezing them, then evaporating the resulting ice, to leave a substantially dry, porous residue which has the same size and shape of the original frozen mass.

Lysate

A product of lysis, which is the disintegration or dissolution of the cell walls.

Lysine

As essential, basic amino acid obtained from many proteins by hydrolysis.

Lysis

The dissolution or destruction of red blood cells, bacteria, or other antigens by a specific lysin (antibody), or by the action of detergents, thus allowing the cell contents to escape.

Lysosome

A membrane-surrounded organelle in the cytoplasm of eukaryotic cells; it contains many hydrolytic enzymes.

M

Machine Welding

Welding with equipment that performs the welding operation under the constant observation and control of a welding operator. The equipment may or may not perform the loading and unloading of the works.

Machine Lines/Process Lines

Surface topography created from machining or honing/ polishing lines will normally run parallel but bisecting (perpendicular) lines may occur when the honing stone mandrel is removed from the work piece.

Macrophage

Large phagocytic cells that are part of the reticuloendothelial system, occurring in the walls of the blood vessels and in loose connective tissue. Usually immobile, macrophages become actively mobile when stimulated by inflammation.

Macromolecules

Molecules whose molecular weights are greater than about 5,000 Daltons.

Macroparticle

Particle with an equivalent diameter greater than 5 µm.

Macrophage

A phagocytic cell of the immune system found in blood and connective tissue and involved in removing debris after injury.

Macroreticular Resin

An ion exchange resin with a reticular porous matrix that makes it effective for removing colloids and bacteria from process streams, as well as dissolved anions. It is especially useful for preventing colloidal and organic fouling of mixed-bed resins and premature clogging of final filters.

Macrorestriction Map

Map depicting the order of and distance between sites at which restriction enzymes cleave chromosomes.

Maintainability

Ease with which maintenance can be performed.

Makeup Air

External air introduced to the air handling system for ventilation and pressurization.

Manual Welding

Welding in which the entire operation is performed and controlled completely by hand.

Manufacture

All operations of receipt of materials, production, packaging, repackaging, labelling, relabelling, quality control, release, storage and distribution of APIs and the related controls.

Manufacturer

The party responsible for the quality of the drug product.

Manufacturing Process

All manufacturing and storage steps in the creation of the finished product from the weighing of components through the storing, packaging, and labeling of the finished product, including, but not limited to, the following: Mixing, granulating, milling, molding, formulating, lyophilizing, tableting, encapsulating, coating, sterilizing, and filling.

Manufacturing Process (Biotechnology)

The basic processes for rDNA fermentation and purification normally include the following steps:

1. Inoculum Preparation: The aim is to develop for the production stage fermentation a pure inoculum in sufficient volume and in the fast-growing (logarithmic) phases so that a high population density is obtained. This is accomplished through a seed fermentation train.
2. The Medium: This is designed to provide the microorganism with all the nutrients it requires. Provision is usually made to add nutrients during fermentation.
3. Oxygen Supply: An adequate supply of oxygen is required. As oxygen is only slightly soluble in water, a number of methods are used to make oxygen more readily available to the microorganisms in the broth, including sparging, mechanical agitators, and dispersion baffles in the fermenter tank.
4. Temperature Control: Heat is generated both by the metabolism of nutrients and by the power dissipated in stirring and has to be removed by controlled cooling. Tank jackets or internal coils are used to control temperature.
5. Antifoam Agents: Microbiological systems that are vigorously stirred and aerated usually produce foam. Excessive foam cannot be tolerated and so provisions have to be made for adding antifoam agents.
6. Harvesting: This is the removal of the cells from the broth. This can be accomplished by cross-flow filtration or centrifugation.
7. Cell Lysis: With E. coli fermentations, the product protein is contained within the cell in the form of an inclusion body. High-pressure homogenizers are often used to chop up the E. coli bacteria into fine fragments, liberating the inclusion bodies for further processing.
8. Purification: This is the separation of the desired product from the other constituents in the harvested broth. Various processes including refolding, ultrafiltration/diafiltration, centrifugation, and chromatographic columns are employed to purify the product.

Marker

An identifiable physical location on a chromosome (e.g., restriction enzyme cutting site, gene) whose inheritance can be monitored. Markers can be expressed regions of DNA (genes) or some segment of DNA with no known coding function but whose pattern of inheritance can be determined.

Marshmallow root (Althea officinalis)

The root soothes mucous membranes; helps heal wounds; ointments and cremes made from the root are effective on chapped hands and lips; internally treats inflammation and problems of the genito-urinary tract; mouthwash; soothes teething pain51.

Mast cells

Cells found in many tissues of the body, which contribute to the allergic and inflammatory process by secreting histamine and other inflammatory particles.

Mastic

Mastic (Pistacia lentiscus) is an evergreen shrub or small tree growing to 3-4 m tall, native to the Mediterranean region from Morocco and Iberia east to Turkey.

A hard, brittle, transparent resin, also known as mastic, is obtained from the tree. The resin is collected by bleeding from small cuts made in the bark.

Mastic flavouring is used for liquors (masticha alcoholic drink) and chewing gum pastiles among other uses. It was the Sultan's privilege to chew mastic, and it was considered to have healing properties.

The best qualities grow in the Greek island of Chios in the Aegean Sea. People in the Mediterranean region have used mastic as a medicine for gastrointestinal ailments for several thousand years. The first century Greek physician and botanist Dioscorides wrote about the medicinal properties of mastic in his classic treatise De Materia Medica ("About Medical Substances").

In recent years, university researchers have provided the scientific evidence for the medicinal properties of mastic. A 1985 study by the University of Thessaloniki discovered that mastic can reduce bacterial plaque in the mouth by 41.5 percent. A 1998 study by the University of Athens found that mastic oil has antibacterial and anti-fungal properties. Another 1998 Nottingham University study published in the New England Journal of Medicine found that mastic can heal pectic ulcers.

Material

A general term used to denote raw materials (starting materials, reagents, process aids, solvents) intermediates, APIs (Active Pharmaceutical Ingredients) and packaging and labelling materials.

Material Containment

The method to incorporate suitable measures into design procedures and operational practices for the containment of materials that can harm personnel and the workplace environment, and minimize potential for cross contamination and housekeeping concerns in the fine chemical, bulk pharmaceutical and pharmaceutical industries. Solids and/or liquids are normally most hazardous in the form of powders and have been divided into the following three categories:

1. Biologically Hazardous additives are compounds that when contacting a living cell, will alter, endanger, or damage the cell in some shape or form. These should be treated as requiring total containment.

2. Chemically Hazardous additives are compounds that when coming into contact with an oxidant, will cause harm to its surroundings due to reaction and/or oxidation. These products usually require containment and/or blanketing with an inert gas.

3. General Intermediates are compounds that are neither biologically nor chemically hazardous additives but they will cause a housekeeping problem. They usually require dusting prevention.

Maximum Cr/Fe Ratio

The maximum ratio of chromium to iron and the depth at which it occurs are the most direct measures of the chromium enrichment in a material oxide layer. Typical ratios are about 1.5 or greater for well-electropolished 316L stainless steel. The depth at which the maximum Cr/Fe ratio is found varies but is usually about one-half the oxide thickness.

Maximum Depth of Enrichment

In stainless steel the chromium enrichment layer comprises all depths at which the chromium concentration is greater than the iron concentration. For well electropolished 316L stainless steel, the maximum depth of this layer is typically 20 to 25 angstroms (Å). Chromium Enrichment Layer Thickness)

Maximum Working Pressure

The pressure at which the system is capable of operating for a sustained period.

Maximum Working Temperature The maximum temperature at which the system may operate for a sustained period. The maximum working temperature should relate to the maximum working pressure and the fluids involved.

Maximum Sustainable Yield

The maximum amount which can be harvested without reducing the stock which is available in subsequent years.

Meadowsweet (Filipendula ulmaria)

Intestinal Astringent, anti-inflammatory, carminative, antacid, anti-emetic. Protects and soothe the mucous membranes of the digestive tract, reducing nausea. It is gentle enough yet its astringency is useful in treating diarrhoea in children.

Mean Kinetic Temperature (MKT)

The single calculated temperature at which the degradation of an article would be equivalent to the actual degradation that results from actual temperature fluctuations during the storage period. It is not a simple arithmetical mean. The MKT is calculated from average storage temperatures recorded over a one-year period, with a minimum of 12 equally spaced storage temperatures being recorded.

Mechanical Completion

The point in a project at which all equipment and materials have been installed, but not commissioned (started-up).

Media (plural of medium)

Substances used to provide sterile nutrients to the fermentation or cell growth process supporting the growth of the live microorganisms. Media may be liquid (broth) or solid, and generally include sucrose or glucose as a carbon source, various minerals, a nitrogen source, and selected growth factors.

Media Prep

The act of preparing nutrient media for cell culture or fermentation.

Medical Devices

Any health care product that does not achieve its principal intended purposes by chemical action in or on the body or by being metabolized. The term "devices" also includes components, parts, or accessories of medical devices, diagnostic aids such as reagents, antibiotic sensitivity disks, and test kits for in vitro diagnosis of diseases and other conditions. There are three classes of medical devices:

1. Class I, General Controls (registration of manufacturers, recordkeeping and labeling requirements, compliance with GMPs).
2. Class II, Special Controls (including performance standards, posmarket surveillance, and patient registries).
3. Class III, Premarket Approval (implanted and life supporting or life sustaining devices).

Medicinal Product

Any substance or combination of substances presented for treating or preventing disease in human beings or animals. Any substance or combination of substances that may be administered to human beings or animals with a view to making a medical diagnosis or to restoring, correcting or modifying physiological functions in human beings or in animals is likewise considered a medicinal product.

Medium (filter)

The material from which a filter is constructed.

Megabase (Mb)

Unit of length for DNA fragments equal to 1 million nucleotides and roughly equal to 1Centimorgan (cM)

Megohm-cm

A measure of ionic purity in water. (also see: Resistivity).

Meiosis

The process of two consecutive cell divisions in the diploid progenitors of sex cells. Meiosis results in four rather than two daughter cells, each with a haploid set of chromosomes.

Melanoma

A cancer that begins in skin cells called melanocytes and spreads to internal organs.

Membrane

A barrier, usually thin, that only permits the passage of particles of a certain size or special nature. Filtration membranes are thin polymer films that are permeable to water and other fluids:

1. Microporous membrane filters have measurable pore structures that physically remove particles or microorganisms larger than pore size.
2. Ultrafiltration membranes (sometimes called molecular sieves) also remove molecules larger than a specified molecular weight.
3. Reverse osmosis membranes are permeable to water molecules and very little else, rejecting even dissolved ions and endotoxins in water.

Menopause

The halt of menstruation of women; usually occurs around the ages of 48 to 50.

Metabolism

The sum of all the physical and chemical reactions, which maintain life processes of an organism. The sum of anabolism, the process by which energy is produced and maintained, and catabolism, the process by which energy is made available to an organism.

2. The sum of the physical and chemical changes in living cells by which energy is provided for vital processes and growth in cell mass.

Metabolite

Any of the various organic compounds produced by metabolism.

Metadata

Electronic records that include processing parameters and audit trail logs. Metadata allows reviewers to replay the original result, or reconstruct a final report from raw data. In chromatography, metadata include integration parameters and calibration tables. An example of metadata can be in long division "1,000 ÷ 5" would be the raw data, the work you had to show on your paper in fourth grade math class would be the metadata, and "200" would be your result.

Metaphase

A stage in mitosis or meiosis during which the chromosomes are aligned along the equatorial plane of the cell.

Metastases

The plural of metastasis.

Metastasis

In cancer, it is the appearance of neoplasms in parts of the body remote from the seat of the primary tumor. It also applies to the transportation of bacteria from one part of the body to another through the blood streams (hematogenous metastasis) or through lymph channels (lymphogenous metastasis).

Methods Validation

Establishing, through documented evidence, a high degree of assurance that an analytical method will consistently yield results that accurately reflect the quality characteristics of the product tested.

Methoxy group

A functional group consisting of an oxygen atom attached to a methyl group ($-OCH_3$).

Methyl Cellulose

A common viscosity-increasing agent used in ophthalmics (also see: Ophthalmic) preparations. It is inversely soluble with temperature.

Methyl group

A functional group consisting of a carbon atom with three hydrogen atoms attached ($-CH_3$).

Mho

Unit of measurement for conductance; the reciprocal of ohm (resistance).

Microbe

A microscopic one-celled organism, animal or vegetable, a microorganism.

Microbiology

The study of microscopic life such as bacteria and viruses.

Microencapsulated

Surrounded by a thin, protective layer of biodegradable substance referred to as microsphere.

Microinch

A unit of length equal to one millionth of an inch (0.000001 inches).

Micron or Micrometer

A unit of length equal to one millionth of a meter (μm) or thousandth of a millimeter (25μm are approximately 0.001 inch.). Bacteria range in size from 0.5μm to 20μm.

Microorganism

A microbe - A microscopic plant or animal, such as a bacterium, protozoan, yeast, virus, or algae.

Microhmo

A measure of conductance equal to one millionth of a mho.

Milk Thistle (Silybum marianum)

Liver protectant, Hepatic, galactogogue, demulcent, cholagogue. Research done in Germany is revealing data about reversal of toxic liver damage as well as protection from potential hepatotoxic agents. As its name implies, it promotes milk secretion in herbal formulas for breast feeding mothers.

Milliequivalent

To simplify the calculation of ion exchange resin capacity, total dissolved ion concentrations are usually converted into equivalent concentrations of calcium carbonate, the most common source of dissolved ions in water. Resin capacity is normally given in ppm as CaCO3, or in grains per gallon as CaCO3 (7,000 grains = 1 pound). However, it may also be given as milliequivalents per liter (meq/L). Since calcium carbonate has a molecular weight of 100 and an equivalent weight of 50 (because calcium has a valence of two) ppm as CaCO3 can be converted to meq/L by dividing by 50. Thus, 1 ppm of CaCO3 = 0.02 meg/L.

Minienvironment

The actual localized control space limited by a defined enclosure that separates or isolates the inside from the outside environment, such that the transfer of potential contamination from one side to the other is minimized or completely eliminated, depending on the design. Minienvironments are not always isolators.

Mitosis

The process of nuclear division in cells that produces daughter cells that are genetically identical to each other and to the parent cell.

Mixed Airflow Room

Room which is supplied of air by conventional "turbulent" means, such as a diffuser or terminal HEPA filter but also includes an unidirectional flow zone (such as a hood over a critical area). Total air changes of the room are greatly enhanced by the operation of the hood.

Mixed-Bed Ion Exchange

Mixing both anion and cation resins in the same deionizer results in higher efficiency, but lower capacity, than separate-bed deionizers.

Moiety

A part or portion of a molecule, generally complex, having a characteristic chemical or pharmacological property.
2. When referring to a molecule, a 'moiety' is a part or section of the whole.

Moist Air

A binary mixture of dry air and water vapor. Each component behaves as if the other is not present and each occupies the complete volume of the mixture.

Molds

Filamentous fungi that have a mycelial structure.

Mole

One gram molecular weight of a compound.

Molecule

A group of atoms arranged to interact in a particular way; one molecule of any substance is the smallest physical unit of that particular substance.

Molecular Genetics

Deals with the study of the nature and biochemistry of genetic material. Includes the technologies of genetic engineering.

Molecular Weight

The weight of a molecule that may be calculated as the sum of the atomic weights of its constituent atoms. Atomic weight is the weight of an element in relation to some element taken as the standard, usually oxygen (16) or carbon (12).

Monamine oxidase

An enzyme that catalyses the oxidation of amines to corresponding aldehydes, ammonia, and hydrogen peroxide.

Monoclonal Antibody (Mab or MoAb)

Antibodies derived from a single source or clone of cells that recognize only one type of antigen. They are produced from hybridomas formed by the hybridization of two cells: a single antibody-producing cell and a cell that can be grown indefinitely in culture (also see: Cell Fusion, Clone, Hybridoma). Monoclonal antibodies have found markets in diagnostic kits and show potential for use in drugs and industrial purification processes.

Monocyte

A mononuclear phagocytic white blood cell derived from the myeloid stem cells. Monocytes circulate in the blood stream and migrate into tissues, where they mature into macrophages.

Monocytes

Large phagocytic leukocytes (white blood cells), which have one nucleus.

Monomer

The basic subunit from which, by repetition of a single reaction, polymers are made. For example, amino acids (monomers) condense to yield polypeptides or proteins (polymers).

Monosaccharides

The building blocks of carbohydrates, hence known as "simple sugar". They are classified by the number of carbon atoms in the molecule, pentoses have five and hexoses six.

Mother Liquor

The residual liquid that remains after the crystallization or isolation processes. A mother liquor may contain unrecovered products (i.e., unreacted starting materials, intermediates, levels of the API and/or impurities). It may be used for further processing.

Motherwort (Leonurus cardiaca)

Antispasm, nervine hepatic, cardiac tonic, hypotensive. The latin names of this plant show its range of uses from delayed menstrual due to anxiety and uterine conditions while cardiaca indicates its use in heart and circulation treatments (due to tension and is often used with Hawthorne berries.

MSDS (Material Safety Data Sheet)

Document describing the chemical and physical properties of a substance as related to its safe handling and storage. The substance manufacturer originates it.

Mucilage

1. A viscid gum dissolved in juices of a plant (natural); 2. In pharmacy, a paste of a gum or dextrin used as an excipient or vehicle (artificial); 3. Or in therapy as a demulcent.

Mucopolysaccharide

A group of polysaccharides containing hexosamine; when dispersed in water form mucins.

Mullein (Verbascum thapsus)

Helps heal respiratory problems52; protects damaged tissue; reduces swelling and pain; has antibiotic qualities53.

Multicellular

Referring to organisms composed of more than one cell - often billions of them, arranged in various organs, tissues, and systems.

Multiplexing

A sequencing approach that uses several pooled samples simultaneously, greatly increasing sequencing speed.

Multi-use Equipment

Equipment used to process more than one product.

Murine

Relating to a member of the rodent family Muridae, including rats and mice; such as murine monoclonal antibodies derived from mice.

Mustard seed

Mustard seeds are small, about 1mm in diameter. They may be coloured from yellowish white to black. They are important spices in many regional cuisines.

In the Indian subcontinent they are often used whole, and are quickly fried in oil until they pop to impart a flavour to the oil.

Mustard oil can be extracted from the seeds. The seeds, particularly the white ones, can also be ground into a flour, and mixed to a thick paste with a little water to make the condiment mustard. The ground mustard powder is usually mixed with ordinary flour to reduce the strength of the resulting condiment.

Other ingredients can be used to mix mustard, for example, sugar, honey, vinegar, wine, or milk.

When initially mixed the sauce is mild in flavour, but it develops in time. Strong mustard has a very powerful (and painful) effect on the nasal membranes if eaten carelessly.

The whole seeds can be soaked in liquid before grinding to create whole grain mustard.

It is possible to buy ready prepared mustard in many places, but the freshly prepared product is usually far superior.

Mutagen

An agent that induces cellular DNA to undergo mutation (e.g. X-rays, mustard gas radiation).

Mutagenic Compounds

Compounds or processes which interact with genetic material directly or indirectly resulting in alteration of the base sequence.

Mutagenesis

The induction of mutation in the genetic material of an organism; researchers may use physical or chemical means to cause mutations that improve the production of capabilities of organisms.

Mutant

The altered cell resulting from mutation of the original wild type or any subsequent alteration.

Mutation

An abrupt change of genotype involving either the structure or number of complete chromosomes or, more commonly, a change in the structure of a single gene so that its function is altered or lost. Certain chemicals called mutagens can induce it.

Myrrh (Balsamodendron myrrha)

Increases mucous membrane activity; helps fight infection by increasing white blood cells (that attack foreign microbials)54; treats weak pulse and cold skin55; stimulates digestion by increasing peptic gland activity; (since myrrh is soothing to mucous membranes, it frequently used in vaginal douches.)

Mycelium

The mat or complex group of protoplasmic units, or the entangled mass of tubelike or filamentous structures, i.e., hyphae, that represents the "body" of plant forms classified as Eumycetes (including Phycomycetes, Ascomycetes, Deuteromycetes (Fungi Imperfectii), and Basidiomycetes).

Mycobacterium

A genus of the family Mycobacteriaceae containing slender, aerobic, usually acid fast, Gram positive, rod-shaped organisms of various forms, club shaped, swollen, but seldom branched or with filaments; it includes many species which were formerly and are still called bacilli, such as the pathogens of tuberculosis and leprosy.

Mycoplasma

The smallest, free-living organism with a size range from 1.25μm to 0.5μm. Pleomorphic (many shapes) because of a lack of a cell wall. Cannot be quantitatively removed by 0.2μm filtration

Myeloma

A malignant human plasma cell that can synthesize excessive amounts of whole antibody or single immunoglobulin chains.

N

National Formulary (NF)

A compendium of purity and testing criteria for chemicals, usually used in combination with the USP.

Native extracts

A viscous, semisolid botanical extract prepared by removing the solvent from a lipid extract.

Necrosis

The pathological death of one or more cells, or of a portion of tissue or organ, resulting from irreversible damage to the nucleus.

NEMA (National Electrical Manufacturers Association)

Enclosures As a way of standardizing enclosure performance, NEMA uses a rating system to identify the enclosure's ability to resist external environmental influences. Resistance to everything from dripping liquid to hose-down to total submersion is defined by this rating system.

1. Type 1 - Enclosures constructed for indoor use to provide a degree of protection to personnel against incidental contact with the enclosed equipment and to provide a degree of protection against falling dirt.
2. Type 2 - Enclosures constructed for indoor use to provide a degree of protection to personnel against incidental contact with the enclosed equipment, to provide a degree of protection

against falling dirt, and to provide a degree of protection against dripping and light splashing of liquids.

3. Type 3 - Enclosures constructed for either indoor or outdoor use to provide a degree of protection to personnel against incidental contact with the enclosed equipment; to provide a degree of protection against falling dirt, rain, sleet, snow, and windblown dust; and that will be undamaged by the external formation of ice on the enclosure.

4. Type 3R - Enclosures constructed for either indoor or outdoor use to provide a degree of protection to personnel against incidental contact with the enclosed equipment; to provide a degree of protection against falling dirt, rain, sleet, and snow; and that will be undamaged by the external formation of ice on the enclosure.

5. Type 3S - Enclosures constructed for either indoor or outdoor use to provide a degree of protection to personnel against incidental contact with the enclosed equipment; to provide a degree of protection against falling dirt, rain, sleet, snow, and windblown dust; and in which the external mechanism(s) remain operable when ice laden.

6. Type 4 - Enclosures constructed for either indoor or outdoor use to provide a degree of protection to personnel against incidental contact with the enclosed equipment; to provide a degree of protection against falling dirt, rain, sleet, snow, and windblown dust, splashing water, and hose-directed water; and that will be undamaged by the external formation of ice on the enclosure.

7. Type 4X - Enclosures constructed for either indoor or outdoor use to provide a degree of protection to personnel against incidental contact with the enclosed equipment; to provide a degree of protection against falling dirt, rain, sleet, snow, and windblown dust, splashing water, hose-directed water, and corrosion; and that will be undamaged by the external formation of ice on the enclosure.

8. Type 5 - Enclosures constructed for indoor use to provide a degree of protection to personnel against incidental contact with the enclosed equipment; to provide a degree of protection against falling dirt; against settling airborne dust, lint, fibers, and flyings; and to provide a degree of protection against dripping and light splashing of liquids.

. Type 6 - Enclosures constructed for either indoor or outdoor use to provide a degree of protection to personnel against incidental contact with the enclosed equipment; to provide a degree of protection against falling dirt; against hose-directed water and the entry of water during occasional temporary submersion at a limited depth; and that will be undamaged by the external formation of ice on the enclosure.

10. Type 6P - Enclosures constructed for either indoor or outdoor use to provide a degree of protection to personnel against incidental contact with the enclosed equipment; to provide a degree of protection against falling dirt; against hose-directed water and the entry of water during prolonged submersion at a limited depth; and that will be undamaged by the external formation of ice on the enclosure

11. Type 12 - Enclosures constructed (without knockouts) for indoor use to provide a degree of protection to personnel against incidental contact with the enclosed equipment; to provide a degree of protection against falling dirt; against circulating dust, lint, fibers, and flyings; and against dripping and light splashing of liquids.

12. Type 12K - Enclosures constructed (with knockouts) for indoor use to provide a degree of protection to personnel against incidental contact with the enclosed equipment; to provide a degree of protection against falling dirt; against circulating dust, lint, fibers, and flyings; and against dripping and light splashing of liquids.

13. Type 13 - Enclosures constructed for indoor use to provide a degree of protection to personnel against incidental contact with the enclosed equipment; to provide a degree of protection against falling dirt; against circulating dust, lint, fibers, and flyings; and against the spraying, splashing, and seepage of water, oil, and noncorrosive coolants.

Neoplasm

Any new growth of cells or tissues but the term is customarily used with rather specific reference to a focus (or a relatively large mass or region) of intermittently or constantly progressive, comparatively unlimited, or uncontrolled new growth that manifests varying degrees of autonomy.

Neem

Neem is obtained from *Azadirachta indica* A Juis (Synonym *Melia Indica).*

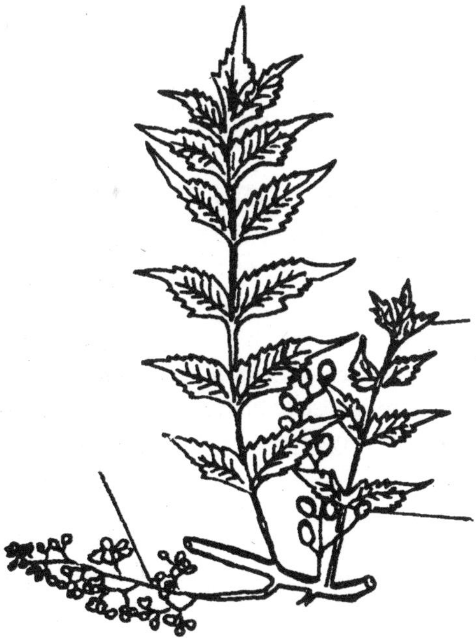

Neem

Nephelometer

Any apparatus used to measure the size and concentration of particles in a liquid by analysis of light transmitted through or reflected by the liquid.

Nephelometry

The semiquantitative estimation of the concentration of particles in a suspension (e.g. bacterial cells in an antigenic preparation), by means of comparing it with the standard suspensions in a nephelometer.

Nephrotoxin
A cytotoxin that is specific for cells of the kidney.

Nettle (Urtica dioaca)
Lactagogue; diuretic and detoxifying; helps heal eczema (especially children when stress related and combined with burdock). As an astrigent in formulas can be used to hlep in uterine hemorrhage.

New Drug Application (NDA)
The New Drug Application contains most of the information included in the IND. Only after FDA approval of the NDA, can distribution and marketing of a new drug begin.

Neuromuscular Junction
The junction between nerve cells and muscle cells. Muscle movement occurs in response to release of the neurotransmitter acetylcholine, by nerve synapses with interface muscle cells.

Neurotransmitter
Substances released from a nerve cell (neuron) at the synapse, the junction that separates nerve cells. The neurotransmitter then travels across the gap to bind to a specific target receptor (usually a large protein molecule embedded in the cell's membrane), to either excite or inhibit it, preventing it from doing so.

Neutrophil
A type of granular leukocyte identifiable by its ease of staining neutral dyes, and by its possession of a nucleus with three to five lobes connected by slender threads of chromatin, and cytoplasm containing fine inconspicuous granules.

Neurotoxic
Destructive to the nerve tissue.

NHSA (Normal Human Serum Albumin)
A blood plasma fraction usually prepared by Cohn cold ethanol precipitation. Dispensed as a 5% to 25% protein solution.

Niche

Role and association of a particular species in the community.

NIH (National Institutes of Health)

Guidelines NIH Guidelines specify practices for constructing and handling recombinant deoxyribonucleic acid (DNA) molecules, and organisms and viruses containing recombinant DNA molecules.

Nitrogenous Base

A nitrogencontaining molecule that has the chemical properties of a base.

NK (natural killer) cells

Large granular lymphocytes (immune cells) that bind to cells and lyse (disrupt) them by releasing cytotoxins (substances toxic to cells).

Nominal (Rating of Filter)

An arbitrary micrometer value indicated by filter manufacturers. Based upon removal of some percentage of particles of a given size or larger, but rarely well defined and consequently not reproducible.

Nominal Pore Size

Based on retention efficiency, a filter should retain 99.9% of particles larger than its nominal rated pore size.

Nominal Outside Diameter

A numerical identification of outside diameter to which tolerances apply.

Nominal Wall Thickness

A numerical identification of wall thickness to which tolerances apply.

Noncarbonate Hardness

Hardness in water caused by chlorides, sulfates, and nitrates of calcium and magnesium.

Non-GMP Technology

Facility design requirement resulting from decisions to address issues outside the realm of GMPs or manufacturer preferences. Often these do affect GMP related design features.

Nonunidirectional Airflow

Air distribution where the first air entering the controlled space mixes with the internal air by means of induction. The airflow that does not meet the definition of unidirectional airflow; previously referred to as "turbulent" or "non-laminar" airflow.

Normal Saline

A very common LVP that has a physiologic (0.9gm%) concentration of sodium chloride.

Northern Blot

A recombinant DNA technique used for the detection of specific RNA transcripts.

Not Exposed or Closed

Drug substance is protected from exposure to the environment during processing.

NPDWR Water

Potable water meeting EPA National Primary Drinking Water Regulations.

Nuclease

An enzyme that breaks down nucleic acids. Exonucleases cleave the nucleotides only at the ends of polynucleotide chains (e.g. phosphodiesterase). Endonucleases attack certain linkates wherever they occur in the polynucleotide chain

Nucleic Acid

A large molecule composed of nucleotide subunits.

Nucleic Acid Hybridization

Matching of either DNA or RNA (depending on the organism)

from an unknown organism with DNA or RNA from a known organism. This method is used in tropical disease research for identifying species and strains of organisms.

Nucleoid

The compact body that contains the genome in a bacterium.

Nucleolus

A discrete region of the nucleus created by the transcription of rRNA genes. The nucleolus disappears during mitosis, or cell division.

Nucleotide

The structural unit of nucleic acids. A subunit of DNA or RNA consisting of purine bases (adenine, guanine), pyrimidine bases (thymine, or cytosine in DNA; uracil, or cytosine in RNA), a phosphate molecule, and a sugar molecule (deoxyribose in DNA and ribose in RNA). Thousands of nucleotides are linked to form a DNA or RNA molecule.

Nucleus

The cellular organelle present in eukaryotes cells and separated from the cytoplasm by a nuclear membrane. It contains the genetic material and is essential for the continued life of the cell.

Object Database Management System (ODBMS)

A database management system specifically designed to manage and store complex objects and their complex relationships; that is, such items are stored as objects rather than as tables or fields. They support modeling and creation of data as objects, allowing for greater flexibility in tracking parent method sets and subcomponents. Such systems may be better than relational database management systems at meeting the data integrity requirements of CFR 21 Part 11.

Nutmeg

The nutmegs *Myristica* are a genus of evergreen trees indigenous to tropical southeast Asia and Australasia. They are important for two spices derived from the fruit, nutmeg and mace.

Nutmeg is the actual seed of the tree, roughly egg-shaped and about 20-30 mm long and 15-18 mm wide, while mace is the dried "lacy" reddish covering of the seed. Several other commercial products are also produced from the trees, including essential oils, extracted oleoresins, and nutmeg butter.

The most important species commercially is the Common or Fragrant Nutmeg Myristica fragrans, native to the Banda Islands of Indonesia; it is also grown in the Caribbean, especially in Grenada. Other species include Papuan Nutmeg M. argentea from New Guinea, and Bombay Nutmeg M. malabarica from India; both are used as adulterants of M. fragrans products.

Nutmeg and mace have similar taste qualities, nutmeg having a slightly sweeter and more delicate flavor. Mace is often preferred in light-coloured dishes for the bright orange, saffron-like colour it imparts.

In Indian cuisine, nutmeg is used almost exclusively in sweets. In European cuisine, nutmeg and mace are used especially in potato dishes and in processed meat products; they are also used in soups, sauces and baked goods.

Japanese varieties of curry powder include nutmeg as an ingredient.

The essential oil is obtained by the steam distillation of ground nutmeg and is used heavily in the perfumery and pharmaceutical industries. The oil is colorless or light yellow and smells and tastes of nutmeg. It contains numerous components of interest to the oleochemical industry, and is used as a natural food flavouring in baked goods, syrups (e.g. Coca Cola), beverages, sweets etc. It replaces ground nutmeg as it leaves no particles in the food. The essential oil is also used in the cosmetic and pharmaceutical industries for instance in tooth paste and as major ingredient in some cough syrups.

In traditional medicine nutmeg and nutmeg oil were used for illnesses related to the nervous and digestive systems. Myristicin in the essential oil is probably the agent responsible for the hallucinogenic properties of nutmeg oil.

Externally, the oil is used for rheumatic pain and, like clove oil, can be applied as an emergency treatment to dull toothache. In France, it is given in drop doses in honey for digestive upsets and used for bad breath. Put 1-2 drops on a cotton swab, and apply to the gums around an aching tooth until dental treatment can be obtained. Use 3-5 drops on a sugar lump or in a teaspoon of honey for nausea, gastroenteritis, chronic diarrhea, and indigestion.

Alternatively a massage oil can be created by diluting 10 drops in 10 ml almond oil. This can be used for muscular pains associated with rheumatism or overexertion. It can also be combined with thyme or rosemary essential oils. To prepare for childbirth, massage the abdomen daily in the three weeks before the baby is due with a mixture of 5 drops nutmeg oil and no more than 5 drops sage oil in 25 ml almond oil.

Nutmeg butter is semi solid and reddish brown in colour. It tastes and smells of nutmeg. Approximately 75% (by weight) of nutmeg butter is trimyristin which can be turned into myristic acid, a 14-carbon fatty acid which can be used as replacement for cocoa butter, can be mixed with other fats like cottonseed oil or palm oil, and has applications as an industrial lubricant.

There is some evidence that Roman priests may have burned nutmeg as a form of incense, although this is disputed. It is known to have been used as a prized and costly spice in the Middle Ages. Saint Theodore the Studite was famous for allowing his monks to sprinkle nutmeg on their pease pudding when required to eat it. In Elizabethan times it was believed that nutmeg could ward off the plague, so nutmeg was very popular. Nutmeg was traded by Arabs during the Middle Ages in the profitable Indian Ocean trade. In the late 15th century, Portugal took over the Indian Ocean trade, including nutmeg, due to the Treaty of Tordesillas with Spain and a separate treaty with the sultan of Ternate. The trade later became dominated by the Dutch in the 17th century.

World production of nutmegs is estimated to average between 10,000 and 12,000 tonnes per year with annual world demand estimated at 9,000 tonnes; production of mace is estimated at 1,500 to 2,000 tonnes. Indonesia and Grenada dominate production and exports of both products with a world market share of 75% and 20% respectively. Other producers include India, Malaysia, Papua New Guinea, Sri Lanka and Caribbean islands such as St. Vincent. The principal import markets are

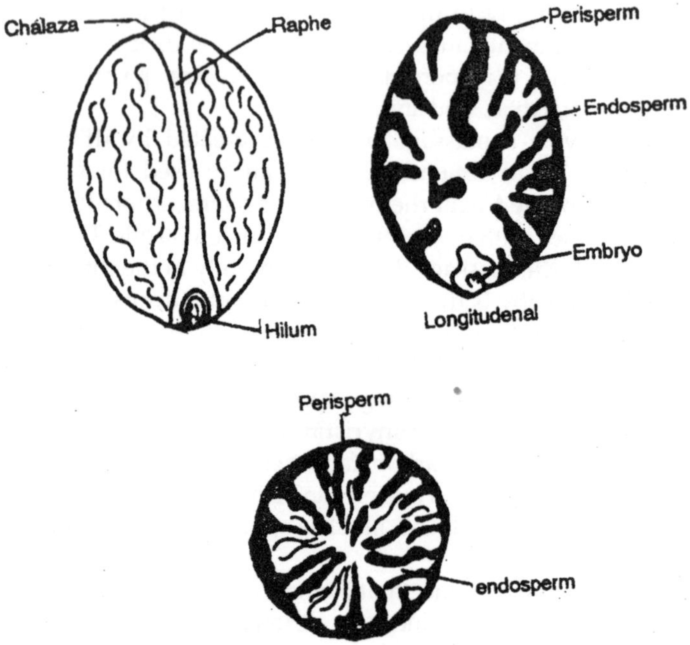

Nutmeg

the European Community, the United States, Japan and India. Singapore and the Netherlands are major re-exporters.

A possible, future use for nutmeg is as a natural control for insects that infest stored cereal grains.

At one time, nutmeg was one of the most valuable spices. It has been said that in England, several hundred years ago, a few nutmeg nuts could be sold for enough money to enable financial independence for life.

The first harvest of nutmeg trees takes place 7-9 years after planting and the trees reach their full potential after 20 years.

In low doses, nutmeg produces no noticeable effect on the body whatsoever. However, at higher doses (10g or more) it is a mild to medium hallucinogen, producing visuals and a comfortable effect almost similar to marijuana. There is a reason this is unpopular, though, as the effects last up to twenty-four hours after the initial peak, (approx. twelve hours after ingestion,) and have unpleasant side effects during the entire process, which linger for up to thirty-six hours. Nutmeg can also cause liver damage if used regularly in large quantities. Nutmeg is extremely toxic when injected intravenously. Excessive consumption of the spice is also dangerous and can lead to death. Nutmeg has in the past been used as an abortifacient, and can also cause hallucinations when taken in excess, along with nausea, dehydration, and generalised body pain, cf. nutmeg psychosis. Large doses (7.5 g or more in a single dose) are dangerous, producing convulsions and palpitations.

Nuxvomica

The drug consists of the seeds of *Strychnos nux-vomica* Linn.

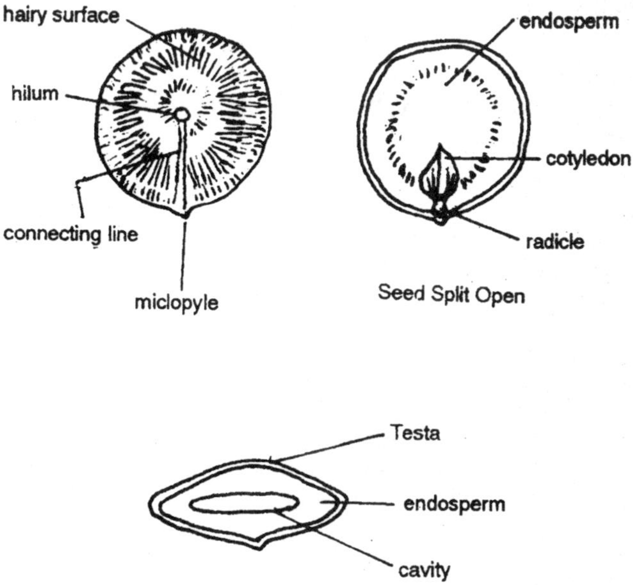

Nuxvomica

O

Oatstraw (Avena sativa)

helps builds the outer layer of the skin; helps detoxify body.

Occupancy

The purpose for which a building or part thereof is used or intended to be used.

Ohm

Unit of electrical resistance in a circuit, such that a potential difference of one volt across a load of one ohm produces a current of one ampere.

Oligomeric

'Oligo' means short. It refers to a type of polymer with only a few subunits, as opposed to a 'monomer' - with one unit, or a 'polymer' - with many subunits. For example, an oligomeric proanthocyanidin is a short-chain polymer consisting of two to four or five flavanol subunits. Oligomers may be further classified as 'dimers' - having two subunits, or 'trimers' - having three subunits.

Oncogene

A gene that when expressed as a protein can lead cells to become cancerous, usually by removing the normal constraints on growth.

Open

Exposed to the environment, not closed.

Open System

A system that fails to meet one or more of the requirements that set the criteria for a closed system.

Operating Parameter

Any information entered into an automated system that is used for automated equipment operation. Or, a parameter indicative of the operating condition of a system.

Operating Range

The validated acceptance criteria within which a control parameter must remain, wherein acceptable product is being manufactured.

Operating System (OS)

The most important program run on a computer because it manages all the other programs. Operating systems perform basic tasks, such as recognizing input from the keyboard, sending output to the display screen, keeping track of files and directories on the disk, and controlling peripheral devices such as disk drives and printers. For large systems, the OS has even greater responsibilities and powers. It regulates traffic, making sure that different programs and users running at the same time do not interfere with each other. The operating system also is responsible for security, ensuring that unauthorized users do not access a system. Microsoft Windows NT, LINUX, and UNIX are operating systems.

Operating Variables

All factors of operation, including control parameters that may potentially affect process state of control and/or fitness for use of the product.

Operation

Room condition when normal process operations are undertaken.

"Operational" Cleanroom

ISO 14644-1 defines "operational" occupancy state as "condition where the installation is functioning in the specified manner, with the specified number of personnel present and working in the manner agreed upon".

Ophthalmic

Of, or relating to the eye, ocular.

Ophthalmics

Pertaining to products for the eyes. GMP requirements for the preparation of ophthalmics are essentially identical to those for parenterals.

Opium

Opium is the latex obtained by making incision on the unripe capsules of *Papaver somniferum* Linn., dried or partly dried by heat or spontaneous evaporation and worked out into some what irregularly shaped massess or moulded into masses of uniform size and shape.

Opportunistic pathogen

Organisms that can cause disease only when the bodily defenses are suppressed.

OQ (Operational Qualification)

Documented verification that aspects of a facility system that can affect product quality perform as intended throughout anticipated operating ranges.

Oral

Relating to the mouth.

Oral Product

A pharmaceutical product meant to be introduced through the mouth in the form of a tablet, capsule, or suspension.

Oral Solid Dosage Drug

Formulated in a solid or powder form for patient to ingest orally.

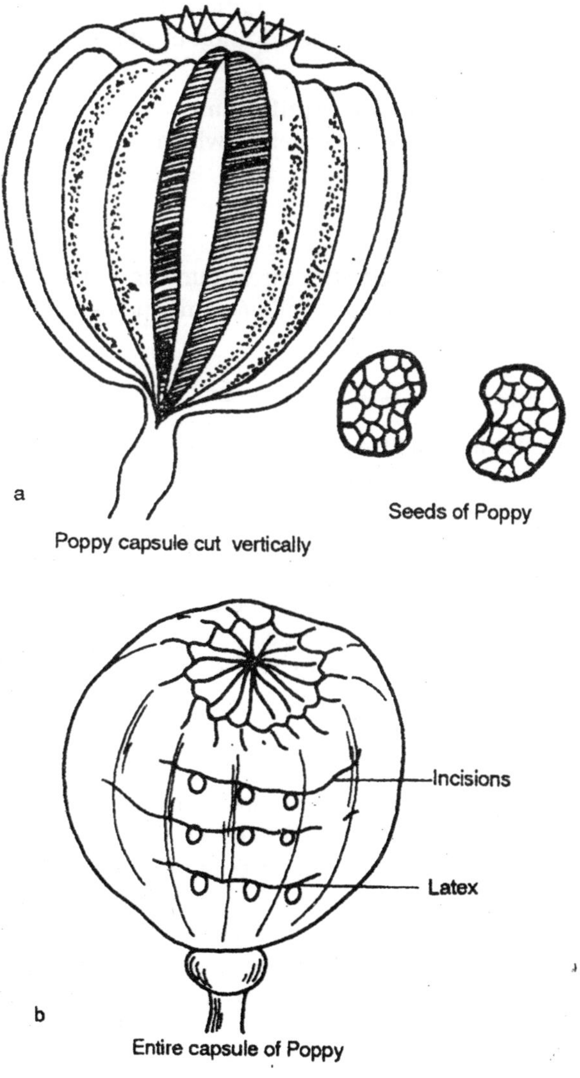
a
Poppy capsule cut vertically
Seeds of Poppy
Incisions
Latex
b
Entire capsule of Poppy

Opium

Orbital Welding

Automatic or machine welding of tubes or pipe in-place with the electrode rotating (or orbiting) around the work. Orbital welding can be done with the addition of filler material or as a fusion process without the addition of filler.

Oregon grape root (Mahonia aquifolium)

Antimicrobial; source of berberine which is an antimicrobial for several bacteria.

Organelles

Membrane-surrounded structures found in eukaryotic cells; they contain enzymes and other components required for specialized cell function.

Organic

Organic matter is a broad category that includes both natural and man-made molecules containing carbon and hydrogen. All living matter in water is made up of organic molecules. The most common are by-products of vegetative decay such as tannins, lignins, and humic acid.

2. In chemistry, any carbon-containing compound (with the exception of molecules like carbon monoxide or carbon dioxide, and materials like graphite and diamonds) is said to be 'organic.'

Organic Peroxide

An organic compound that contains the bivalent -0-0- structure and which may be considered to be a structural derivative of hydrogen peroxide where on or both of the hydrogen atoms have been replaced by an organic radical. Organic peroxides can present an explosion hazard (detonation or deflagration) or they can be shock sensitive. They can also decompose into various unstable compounds over an extended period.

Organism

A single, autonomous living thing. Bacteria and yeasts are organisms; mammalian and insect cells used in culture are not.

Organosulfur

An organic compound containing sulfur.

Origin

Point or region where DNA replication is begun. Often abbreviated Ori.

Orphan Drug

The FDA grants Orphan Drug status to one company for a drug that is believed to substantially increase the life expectancy of the treated patient for a particular disease. This excludes other companies from receiving an FDA license to produce a similar drug for a finite period (usually 7 years), thereby allowing the company producing the drug to recuperate their R&D expenses.

Osha root (Ligusticum porteri)

Reduces inflammation of the throat and mucous membranes; increases elimination of toxins throughout the spores of the skin; acts like a bronchial dilator.

Osmosis

The diffusion of a solvent through a semipermeable membrane from a solution of higher concentration to one of lower concentration until there are equal concentrations of fluid on both sides of the membrane.

Osmotic Pressure

Pressure generated by the osmotic flow of water through a membrane into a (aqueous) phase containing a solute in a higher concentration.

Osteoporosis

A disease process that results in a reduction in bone mass per unit volume. Bone loss is a universal process of aging, but occurs at an accelerated rate in women past menopause.

Out of Specification

An examination, measurement, or test result that does not comply with preestablished criteria.

Oxidation (on metals)

The formation of an oxide layer on a metal surface. When oxidation occurs because of welding, it is visible as discoloration. The discoloration or heat tint produced by oxidation has been associated with the onset of corrosion in stainless steel piping systems.

Oxidation/Reduction

In phytochemistry, you can think of 'oxidation' as adding an atom of oxygen or removing an atom of hydrogen from a molecule. You can think of 'reduction' as removing an oxygen atom or adding a hydrogen atom to a molecule.

Oxide Thickness

The depth at which the oxide signal has fallen to half the maximum peak height. Typical values for well electropolished 316L stainless steel range from 20 to 50 angstroms (Å).

Oxide Layer

In welding, an area usually located in the heat-affected zone (HAZ) of the weldment where an oxidation reaction has taken place.

Oxidizer

A material other than a blasting agent or explosive, that readily yields oxygen or other oxidizing gas, or that readily reacts to promote or initiate combustion of combustible materials. Oxidizers are subdivided as follows:

1. Class 4 - An oxidizer that can undergo an explosive reaction due to contamination or exposure to thermal or physical shock. In addition, the oxidizer will enhance the burning rate and may cause spontaneous ignition of combustible materials.
2. Class 3 - An oxidizer that will cause a severe increase in the burning rate of combustible materials with which it comes in contact or that will undergo vigorous, self-sustained decomposition due to contamination or exposure to heat.
3. Class 2 - An oxidizer that will cause a moderate increase in the burning rate or that may cause spontaneous ignition of combustible materials with which it comes in contact.

4. Class 1 - An oxidizer whose primary hazard is that it slightly increases the burning rate but does not cause spontaneous ignition when it comes in contact with combustible materials.

Ozone

Formed by an electric discharge or by the slow combustion of phosphorus, ozone is a modified and condensed form of oxygen, in which three atoms of oxygen are combined to form the molecule, O3. Because it is a powerful oxidizing agent it is used in deionized water systems to kill bacteria and to reduce by oxidation the amount of Total Organic Carbon (TOC) in the water. Air containing a perceptible amount of ozone has an odor suggesting chlorine or sulfurous acid gas.

P

Packaged Equipment

An assembly of individual pieces or stages of equipment, complete with inter-connecting piping and connections for external piping. The assembly may be mounted on a skid or other structure prior to delivery.

Packaging

All operations, including filling and labeling, which a bulk product has to undergo in order to become a finished product.

Packaging Material

Any material intended to protect an intermediate or API (Active Pharmaceutical Ingredient) during storage and transport.

Pandemic Disease

An epidemic over an especially wide geographic area.

Paprika

Paprika is a sweet-to-mildly hot cultivar of the chile pepper (Capsicum annuum, of the family Solanaceae). Paprika peppers are elongated or round fruit, bright red, yellow or green.

Paprika plants tolerate nearly every climate and are grown all over the world. A fairly warm climate is necessary for a strong aroma.

Hungary is probably the world's leading producer of paprika. In fact, the Hungarian word "paprika" refers not only to this type of pepper, but to all peppers in general. (Prompted by the discovery of high levels of potential carcinogenic aflatoxins in its popular spice, Hungary banned sales of the ingredient in October 2004, though it has since resumed sales in a more supervised manner.)

In the United States, California and Texas are the main producers.

Paprika is often eaten as a ground powder but sometimes as a fresh vegetable. It is commonly used in Hungarian, Balkan, Middle Eastern, and Central Asian cuisines. The round type can be stuffed with cottage cheese or salad to make a portable lunch.

Small slices of pickled paprika are traditionally stuffed into green olives in the U.S. — see pimento.

Some specialty varieties of paprika are hot but the generally available ground preparation is quite mild.

PAR (Proven Acceptable Range)

A range for a critical parameter that has been determined to be achievable and appropriate for the process or processes with which it is associated. It is established by knowledge gained through relevant documentation and actual testing. A process should perform consistently and as intended when all critical parameters are held within the established PARs.

Parent compound

A compound from which other compounds are derived. For example, alliin is the parent compound of allicin.

Parenteral Drug (LVP, SVP)

A parenteral drug is defined as one intended for injection through the skin or other external boundary tissue, rather than through the alimentary canal, so that active substances they contain are administered, using gravity or force, directly into a blood vessel, organ, tissue, or lesion. They are infused when administered intravenously (IV), or injected when administered intramuscularly (IM), or subcutaneously into the human body. A large volume parenteral (LVP) is a unit dose container of greater than 100ml that is terminally sterilized by heat. Small volume parenteral (SVP) is a "catch-all" for all non-LVP parenterals products except biologicals.

Particle

Solid or liquid object which for purposes of classification of air cleanliness, falls within a cumulative distribution that is based upon a threshold (lower limit) size in the range from 0,1 µm to 5 µm.

Particle Size

The apparent maximum linear dimension of a particle in the plane of observation as seen with a microscope or the equivalent diameter of a particle detected by automatic instrumentation. The equivalent diameter is the diameter of a reference sphere having known properties and producing the same response in the sensing instrument as the particle being measured.

Particle Concentration

Number of individual particles per unit volume of air.

Particulate Usually a solid particle large enough to be removed by filtration. Nonfilterable solids are usually referred to as colloids.

Passion flower (Passiflora incarnata)

Sedative56; assists relaxation and sleep.

Passive Immunity

Temporary immunity produced by administration of gamma globulin.

Passivity

The state in which a stainless steel exhibits a very low corrosion rate. Also known as passivity, is the loss (or minimizing) of chemical reactivity exhibited by certain metals and alloys under special environmental conditions.

Passivation

A final chemical treatment/cleaning process that removes exogenous iron or iron compounds from the surface of stainless steel piping and equipment by the use of a mild oxidant, such as a nitric acid solution, or by "in-situ electropolishing. The purpose of passivation is to restore and/or enhance the spontaneous formation of the chemically inert surface or protective passive film.

Passive Layer

A passive oxidized film that forms naturally on a stainless steel surface when exposed to air or similar oxidizing environment thus protecting the underlying base metal from corrosion. Welding disturbs the passive layer by reducing the chromium and increasing the iron, thus altering the chromium/iron ratio (measure of corrosion resistance). Upon completion and approval of the weld, the weld surface and adjacent boundary area must be brought back to a passive state. Additionally, normal operating conditions in typical Water For Injection, reverse osmosis, deionized water, clean steam, Clean In Place, and process piping often lead to formation of the most prevalent form of self catalyzing corrosion called "rouge" (French for red), which is a colloidal form of rust containing iron oxide, chromium and nickel in various forms. This problem is further accentuated by high temperature. The rouge layer acts as a passive layer until it becomes so thick that it "sloughs off" into the process or water stream.

Pasteurization

The heating of milk, wines, fruit juices, etc., for about thirty minutes at 68°C (154.4°F) whereby the living bacteria are destroyed, but the flavor or bouquet is preserved; the spores are unaffected, but are kept from developing by immediately cooling the liquid to 10°C (50°F) or lower.

Pathogen

An organism (including viruses, virions and prions) capable of causing disease.

2. A micro-organism or substance capable of producing disease.

3. Any microbiological or eukaryotic cell containing sufficient genetic information, which upon expression of such information is capable of producing disease in healthy people, plants, or animals.

Pathogenic

Causing or capable of causing disease.

Pathogenic Organisms

Organisms capable of causing disease, either directly (by infecting) or indirectly (by producing a toxin that causes illness).

Pau D'Arco (Tabebuia impetiginosa)

Retards the development of tumors; helps heal candida in adults thrush (candida in the infant's mouth); helps heal viruses; anti-fungal; assists in eliminating parasites. Dr. T. Meyer learned from the Callaway tribe and using it on his leukemia patients with success. In 1960, it's use was taken up by the Municipal Hospital of Santo Andre where medical doctors used a brew of the bark on terminal cancer patients that helped them with pain and reduction o the size of the tumors.

PE (Polyethylene)

A thermoplastic material that varies from type to type according to the particular molecular structure of each type, i.e. its crystallinity, molecular weight, and molecular weight distribution. These variations are possible through changes in polymerization conditions used during manufacturing. Low-density polyethylene (LDPE) has a melt point of 221°F (105°C), specific gravity of 0.91 to 0.925 g/cc, increased toughness, stress cracking resistance, clarity, flexibility, and elongation. It also has reduced creep and mold shrinkage. Polyethylene of higher density such as HDPE has better permeation barrier properties, hardness, abrasion resistance, chemical resistance, and surface gloss. It is important to note that photo or light oxidation will occur when natural PE is exposed to UV radiation, usually from the sun.

Penetrance

A term indicating the likelihood that a given gene will actually result in disease.

Penicillin

An antibiotic containing a ß-lactam ring that inhibits an enzyme responsible for making peptide cross-links in the bacterial cell wall. It is obtained from cultures of the molds Penicillium Notatum or Penicillium Chrysogenum.

Penicillium

The genus of mold causing a zone of inhibition in an agar plate of bacteria. It is the organism, which produces natural penicillin.

Peptide A secondary protein derivative defined as "a definitely characterized combination of two or more amino acids, the carboxyl (COOH) group of one being united with the amino (NH2) group of the other, with the elimination of a molecule of water". They form a peptide bond.

Peppermint (Mentha piperita)

Reduces cramps, antispasm, stimulant.

Pepper

There are several completely different plants referred to by the name of pepper; most are used in food for the "hot" sensation that particular chemical components induce on the tongue.

1. Various plants in the family Piperaceae, notably the genus Piper, including the black pepper that appears on virtually every dining room table in parts of the world. Different preparations of the same Piper nigrum plant also produce "white" and "green" peppercorns. Also, the genus Peperomia, which is included in the Peperomiaceae family by some authors.
2. Plants in the genus Capsicum in the family Solanaceae, including bell peppers and chile peppers. These plants have given rise to the Scoville scale to measure the "hotness" of a pepper.
3. Pink peppercorns, also called "Peruvian pepper" or "Caribbean pepper," are from a plant related to Cashews; species Schinus molle, in the family Anacardiaceae.
4. Szechuan peppercorns are produced by a plant of the family Rutaceae, species Zanthoxylum piperitum.

Peptide Hormones

A diverse class of hormones that are synthesized and excreted at various sites within the body. Examples include: insulin, relaxin, glucagons, growth hormone, vasopressin, ACTH (Adrenocorticotropic Hormone), endorphins, and encephalins.

Percent Rejection

In reverse osmosis or ultrafiltration, the ratio of impurities removed to total impurities in the incoming feedwater. For example, RO membranes typically remove (reject) 90% of the dissolved inorganic contaminants in water.

Peri menopause

The years of a women's life immediately preceding menopause.

Peristalsis

A progressive, wavelike movement that occurs involuntarily in hollow tubes of the body, esp. the alimentary canal.

Peristaltic Pump

A type of positive displacement pump that operates by pulsations of flow caused by passing rollers over flexible tubing. Operating pressure limited by tubing tolerance.

Permeability

he ability of a body to pass a fluid under pressure.
Permeate In reverse osmosis, the water that diffuses through the membrane, thereby becoming purified water.

Permissible Exposure Limit (PEL)

The maximum permitted eight-hour time-weighted average concentration of an airborne contaminant.

Permissions or Privileges

Security codes that define or restrict which users can read, write, and execute the associated files, directories, or programs. Some departments need to look only at data, some need to input data or run programs, and others may not need to look at the data at all.

Peroxisome

Very small membrane-bound particles responsible for photorespiration in plants. Similar to lysosome in structure, but not in function.

Petrolatum

White petrolatum is a purified mixture of semi-solid hydrocarbons obtained from petroleum. It is a common base or carrier for ointments. It can be sterile filtered at elevated temperatures.

pH

Chemistry: potential hydrogen. A scale of expressing the acidity or alkalinity of a substance; maximum acidity is pH 0 and maximum alkalinity is pH 14. The scale is logarithmic, thus there is a ten-fold difference between pH units.

2. The pH value of an aqueous solution is a number describing its acidity or alkalinity. A pH is the negative logarithm (base 10) of the concentration of hydrogen ions (equivalent per liter). The pH value of a neutral solution is 7. An acidic solution has a pH less than 7, while a basic solution has a pH greater than 7, up to 14.

3. A measure of the acidity or alkalinity of a substance. Neutral pH (pure water) is 7; acidic is less than 7 and basic, or alkaline, is above 7. Examples: vinegar, 2.4-3.4; stomach acid, 1.0-3.0; blood, 7.4; baking soda, 8.4.

Phage

A virus for which the natural host is a bacterial cell. (also see: Bacteriophage)

Phagocyte A cell that engulfs foreign particles from its surroundings by a process called phagocytosis. The cell releases hydrolytic enzymes from intracellular bodies called lysosomes that partially digest the foreign particle, after which it is further degraded in the phagocyte cytoplasm.

Phagocytosis

Ingestion and digestion of bacteria by phagocytes.

Pharmaceutical

A medicinal drug, or relating to or engaged in pharmacy or the manufacture and sale of pharmaceuticals. A pharmaceutical product is generally one that is made up using available chemical compounds.

Pharmaceutical Area

A general manufacturing area classification designated by the need for a change of clothing (e.g., Packing Hall). See ISPE® Sterile Baseline Guide.

Pharmacodynamics

The study of the physiological effects and mechanisms of action of a compound and how this varies with concentration/ dosage. In other words, the study of how the drug acts upon the body.

Pharmacognosy

1. An applied science which deals with the biologic, biochemical, and economic features of natural drugs and their constituents. It is the study of drugs having their origin in the plant and animal kingdom.
2. The study of natural drugs and their physical, botanical, pharmacological, and chemical properties.
3. The study of medicinal plants and their extracts, constituents, and phytochemistry. Pharmacognosy (from the Greek words for drug or medicine and knowledge) is currently considered to be a branch of pharmacology and is studied in schools of pharmacy.

Pharmacokinetics

Study of the metabolism and action of drugs with particular emphasis on their absorption, excretion, and duration of action.
2. The study of how compounds are absorbed, distributed, metabolized and eliminated by the body. In other words, the study of how the body acts upon the drug.

Phenolic

A molecule containing an aromatic ring that bears one or more hydroxyl groups is referred to as 'phenolic.' Examples include flavonoids, isoflavonoids, and lignans. The word comes from 'phenol,' the name for the structure below which has one hydroxyl group attached to the ring.

Phenols

Phenols, which are also called polyphenols or phenolic compounds, are plant substances which have an aromatic ring bearing one or more hydroxyl groups (Harborne and Baxter, 324). Phenols are widely splattered throughout the plant kingdom. Food and drink owe their actions on our senses to phenols. To many other phytochemical classifications this is the parent group, but phenols may also be contained as constituents in compounds through which a botanical phytochemical exists under a different classification.

The flavonoids constitute about one-half of the eight-thousand or so recognized phenols. The rest are broken down into phenylpropanoids, anthones, stilbenoids, and quinones. The compounds have a myriad of medical functions. From the perspective of the plant kingdom, polyphenolic compounds are important contributors to the survival of plant species through the insurance of successful pollination, and also provide plants with an unpleasant taste so that possibly threatening herbivores are repelled.

Flavonoids are molecules responsible for the color of fruit and flowers. They are beneficial to man as powerful antioxidants, stress modifiers, anti-allergic agents, anti-viral compounds and anti-carcinogens. Some are able to stimulate protein synthesis, and some are known antiinflammatory agents. Still others have demonstrated vaso-protective activity. Some are diuretic, antispasmodic, antibacterial,and antifunga.

While some flavonoids may be classified as flavonoid glycosides, all are phenols, but flavonoids, flavonals, flavanones, isoflavones, and xanthones, all stem from flavones. Flavones have effectively been used to tone blood cell walls and bloodcells. Anthocyanidins and anthocyanins are related flavonoids. These, and flavones in general, occur most frequently as glycosides.

Isoflavones occur less frequently as glycosides, more often in their free state, and have a higher degree of structural variation.

Tannins are polyphenolic compounds and are divided into

two groups, i.e., the hydrolyzable and non-hydrolyzable tannins, and the condensed tannins. Hydrolyzable tannins are thought to be hepatotoxic with overuse; condensed tannins appear not to have this action.

In general, tannins are astringent and antiseptic. Hamamelitannin, from witch hazel bark is a source of pharmacologically-used tannin (Evans, 386-388) and often found in men's aftershave lotions. A polyphenol classified as a napthaquinone, plumbagin, for example, found in the Round Leaved Sundew (Drosera rotundifolia) a plant indigenous to coastal Maine, has shown anti-bacterial properties and continues to be researched for its anti-cancer actions.

2. An organic acid often used as a disinfectant. Proper strength for a bacteriocidal preparation is 5%. Sometimes dispersed as an aerosol "fog" in manufacturing rooms.

Phospholipid

A lipid substance containing phosphorous, fatty acids, and nitrogenous base.

Photoautotrophs

Facultative autotrophs that obtain their energy from light.

Photoluminescent

The property of emitting light as the result of absorption of visible or invisible light, which continues for a length of time after excitation.

Photo Oxidation

The mechanism by which ultraviolet light reduces Total Organic Carbon (TOC) to Carbon Dioxide. If halogenated organics are present, both CO2 and mineral acids can be formed.

Phycomycetes Algalike fungi that do not posses chlorophyll and cannot photosynthesize. Aquatic and terrestrial molds belong to this category.

Photosensitisation

Condition in which the skin reacts abnormally to light,

especially to ultraviolet radiation or sunlight. Cause by the presence of drugs, hormones, or heavy metals in the system.

Physical Barrier

Any equipment, facilities, or devices (e.g., fermentors, factories, filters, thermal oxidizers) that are designed to achieve containment.

Physical Hazard

A classification of a chemical for which there is scientifically valid evidence that it is a combustible liquid, compressed gas, cryogenic, explosive, flammable gas, flammable liquid, flammable solid, organic peroxide, oxidizer, pyrophoric, unstable, (reactive), or water-reactive material.

Physical Manipulation

A process other than a chemical reaction that may change the purity of the physical properties of the material, including but not limited to, crystallization, recrystallization, gel filtration, chromatography, milling, drying, or blending.

Physical Map

A map of the locations of identifiable landmarks on DNA (e.g., restriction enzyme cutting sites, genes), regardless of inheritance. Distance is measured in base pairs. For the human genome, the lowest-resolution physical map is the banding patterns on the 24 different chromosomes; the highest resolution map would be the complete nucleotide sequence of the chromosomes.

Physiology

The study of the functions of living organisms and the chemical and physical processes, which are involved in living systems.

Physiological concentrations

Concentrations of a substance likely to occur within the human body. Results from research that uses significantly higher or lower concentrations of the chemical being studied may not be applicable to the actual situation inside the body.

Phytoalexin

An antimicrobial, protective compound synthesized by a plant in response to bacterial, viral, or fungal infection. Many chemicals that are medicinal to humans are phytoalexins.

Phytochemistry

The branch of chemistry that focuses on the constituents of plants (phyto comes from the Greek word for plant). Often, phytochemistry deals specifically with the chemistry of medicinal plants. This discipline can also include studies of how to extract, concentrate, analyze, standardize, & preserve herbal products.

Phytoestrogen

A plant constituent, which displays estrogenic activity.

Phytophamaceutical

A pharmaceutical or medicinal preparation derived from a plant.

Picrorhiza

It consist of dried roots and rhizomes of *Picrorhiza kurroa.* Royale ex Benth.

Pipe Size

Pipe size is determined by diameter and schedule. For bioprocessing equipment, pipe does not include tube.

Pit

A small surface void resulting from a localized loss of base metal by corrosion or etching, or by the removal of surface inclusions during electropolishing or passivation. A pit may or may not be detectable during liquid penetrant inspection.

Pitch

To cause to be set at a particular angle or slope. Degree of slope or elevation.

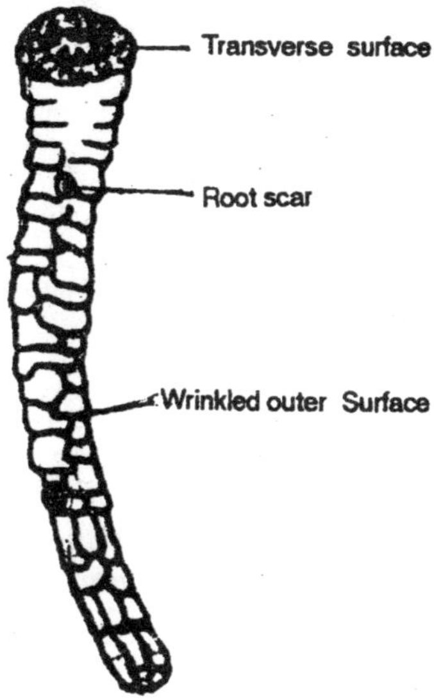

Picrorhiza

Pituitary

Endocrine gland attached to the bottom surface of the hypothalamus, which secretes hormones that regulate a number of functions including metabolism, growth and reproduction. Often referred to as the "master gland of the body."

Placebo

An inactive substance given to satisfy a patient's desire for medication, or used as an inactive control in controlled studies of drug actions.

2. An inert or innocuous substance used in controlled experiments testing the efficacy of another substance.

Plankton

Those microorganisms that are passively floating or drifting in a body of water.

Plaque

A clear zone in a bacterial culture grown on an agar plate caused by localized destruction of bacterial cells by a bacteriophage. Applying the fluid to a culture and counting the number of plaques formed can estimate the concentration of infective virus in a fluid.

Plantain (Plantago ovaga)

Alleviates skin infection and inflammation57; also reduces pain and coughing58.

Plasma

The liquid portion of blood in which the cellular elements are suspended. As a fresh liquid obtained by centrifugation, plasma is a clear, amber-colored solution containing eight to nine percent solids; of these, 85 percent are proteins while the other components are the lipids, which include the neutral fats, fatty acids, lecithin, and cholesterol. Also present are sodium, chloride and bicarbonate, potassium, calcium and magnesium. A most essential function of plasma is the maintenance of blood pressure and the exchange with tissue of nutrients for waste. Contains fibrinogen.

Plasma Cell

A cell derived from a B-lymphocyte and solely responsible for the production of antibodies. Each plasma cell forms only one type of antibody and is characterized by an eccentric nucleus, a prominent Golgi zone, bulky basophilic cytoplasm (due to an extensive endoplasmic reticulum) and large numbers of mitochondria.

Plasma Membrane

The physical barrier that surrounds the cytoplasm of all cells. It is composed of lipid, protein, and carbohydrate and is semi-permeable.

Plasma Proteins

The proteins found in plasma, usually divided into albumin, globulin and fibrinogen fractions.

Plasmid

Self-replicating, extrachromosomal circular DNA molecules, distinct from the normal bacterial genome and nonessential for the cell survival under nonselective conditions. Some plasmids are capable of integrating into the host genome. A number of artificially constructed plasmids are used as cloning vectors.

Plastics

High molecular weight polymers or copolymers. The wide range in physical properties of polymeric materials allows for utilization as elastomers, fibers, adhesives, rigid castings, composites, and laminates. ASTM D883 defines a plastic as a material that contains as an essential ingredient, one or more organic polymeric substances of large molecular weight, is solid in its finished state, and, at some stage in its manufacture into finished articles, can be shaped by flow. Plastics, or more appropriately polymers, are composed primarily of carbon, hydrogen, oxygen, silicon, chlorine, fluorine, and nitrogen, in various combinations and permutations. Plastics are grouped into two categories: 1. Thermoplastics: can be melted, cooled and remelted without destroying the physical or mechanical characteristics of the polymer. This property permits components to be molded or extruded. Thermoplastic polymers include: Chlorinated Vinyls, Fluorinated plastics, Ketone, Nitrile, Nylon, Polyamide-imide, Polyolefin, Polycarbonate, and Acrylonitrile butadiene styrene (ABS). (also see: Chlorinated Vinyls, Fluorinated Plastics, Polyolefin) 2. Thermosets: begin as a liquid or powder that through chemical reaction with a second reactant or through catalyzed polymerization result in anew product with characteristics different from either starting material. Thermoset resins include: Epoxy, Phenolic, Polyurethane, Silicone, Urea and Melamine, Polyester, Vinyl ester, Furan, Bisphenol A fumarate.

Plastics, U.S.P. Classification

(also see: Biological Reactivity Tests, In Vivo)

Platelet

A round or oval disc, 2 to 4 microns in diameter, lacking

hemoglobin, found in the blood of vertebrates. Platelets play an important role in blood coagulation, hemostasis, and blood thrombin formation; syn: thrombocyte.

Platelet activating factor (PAF)

A hormone that activates platelets to secrete serotonin and other mediators to cause smooth muscle contraction and increase vascular permeability, reactions, which are important in asthma.

PLC (Programmable Logic Controller)

An automated system with analog capability as well as binary (discrete). PLCs must be equipped with a digital interface to a "front end" computer for data collection and for programmer interface.

PLC Controlled Automated System

Any automated system using a Programmable Logic Controller as its primary controller.

Plena

The plural of plenum.

Plenum

An enclosure in which air or other gas is at a pressure greater than that outside the enclosure.

Pleurisy root (Asclepias tuberosa)

Remedy for colds and flus; expectorant.

Pleuropneumonia

A specific infectious disease in cattle characterized by inflammation of the lung and pleura, generally called contagious pleuropneumonia. It is due to a virus.

Poison

Any substance which when taken into the body in a single dose of 1.0 gm. or less, is injurious to health or dangerous to life.

Polyalphaolefin (PAO)

A synthetic oil used in lieu of DOP for HEPA filter testing.

Polygenic Disorder

Genetic disorder resulting from the combined action of alleles of more than one gene (e.g., heart disease, diabetes, and some cancers). Although such disorders are inherited, they depend on the simultaneous presence of several alleles; thus the hereditary patterns are usually more complex than those of single gene disorders.

Polyhydroxylated

A molecule bearing more than one hydroxyl group is called polyhydroxylated.

Polymer

A large molecule consisting of a number of identical or similar subunits joined together. An example is the starch molecule, which is made up of numerous glucose units. Proteins can be thought of as polymers of amino acid units. Lignin, the polymer that gives wood its rigidity, is a polymer of cinnamyl alcohol units (lignans are made of two joined cinnamyl alcohols).

Polyolefin

The polyolefin polymer is probably one of the most economical and widely used classes of thermoplastics, including such materials as PB, PP, and PE. PB is a semicrystalline polymer based on polybutene, homopolymers, and either polybutene or polyethylene copolymers. The primary use of PB is pipe with hydrostatic pressure rating of 1,000 psi at 73°F. PP is a crystalline polymer that has good resistance to caustics, solvents, acids, and other organic chemicals, but is not resistant to oxidizing-type acids, detergents, alcohols, or chlorinated organic materials. It is suitable for pipe applications. The largest group of polyolefins is linear PE. It includes ULDPE, LLDPE, LDPE, HDPE, HMW-HDPE, and UHMWPE. These density descriptions generally refer to ASTM designations based on unmodified polymers. PE types of higher density have better permeation barrier properties, hardness, abrasion resistance, chemical resistance, and higher surface gloss.

Polished Water

High purity water after it has undergone a second treatment step. Ultrapure water usually undergoes two or more treatment steps. More economical pretreatment processes (e. g., reverse osmosis) are used to remove all but a very small fraction of the impurities. Highly efficient polishing processes (e. g., mixed-bed deionization) are used to remove the impurities that remain.

Polymer

A macromolecule (long chain) consisting of five or more repeating units called monomers. Examples include polyethylene, polystyrene, and PTFE (polytetrafluoroethylene).

Polymerase

An enzyme that catalyzes production of nucleic acid molecules.

Polymerase Chain Reaction (PCR)

A method for amplifying a DNA base sequence using a heatstable polymerase and two 20-base primers, one complementary to the (+) strand at one end of the sequence to be amplified and the other complementary to the (-) strand at the other end. Because the newly synthesized DNA strands can subsequently serve as additional templates for the same primer sequences, successive rounds of primer annealing, strand elongation, and dissociation produce rapid and highly specific amplification of the desired sequence. PCR also can be used to detect the existence of the defined sequence in a DNA sample.

Polymorphism

Difference in DNA sequence among individuals. Genetic variations occurring in more than 1% of a population would be considered useful polymorphisms for genetic linkage analysis. (also see: Mutation

Polypeptide

A long chain of amino acids covalently bound by peptide.

Pomegranate

The pomegranate Punica granatum is a species of fruit-bearing deciduous shrub or small tree growing to 5-8 m tall. Although it was previously given its own family Punicaceae, recent genetic evidence shows that it is a member of the family Lythraceae. The pomegranate is believed to have originated in the area from Iran east to northern India, but has been cultivated around the Mediterranean for so long (several millennia) that its true native range is not accurately known. The genus name, Punica is named after the Phoenicians, who were active in spreading its cultivation, partly for religious reasons. Its species name granatum derives from the Latin adjective granatus, meaning 'granular'. The city of Granada in Spain became an early centre of cultivation, and was named after the fruit.

The leaves are opposite or sub-opposite, glossy, narrow oblong, entire, 3-7 cm long and 2 cm broad. The flowers are bright red, 3 cm diameter, with five petals (often more on cultivated plants). The fruit is between an orange and a grapefruit in size, 7-12 cm diameter, has a thick reddish skin and many seeds. The edible part is the brilliant red seed pulp surrounding the seeds.

The only other species in the genus, Socotra Pomegranate Punica protopunica, is endemic on the island of Socotra. It differs in having pink (not red) flowers and smaller, less sweet fruit.

Pomegranates are drought tolerant, and can be grown in dry areas with either a Mediterranean winter rainfall climate or in summer rainfall climates. In wetter areas, they are prone to root decay from fungal diseases. They are tolerant of moderate frost, down to about -10°C.

The arils (seed casings) of the pomegranate are consumed raw. The entire seed is eaten, though the fleshy outer portion of the seed is the part that is desired. The taste differs depending on the variety of pomegranate and its state of ripeness. It can be very sweet or it can be very sour or tangy, but most fruits lie somewhere in between, which is the characteristic taste.

The acidic juice of pomegranates is used in Indian cookery; thickened and sweetened it makes grenadine syrup, used in cocktail mixing. The juice can also be used as an antiseptic when applied to cuts.

Pomegranate seeds are sometimes used as a spice.

Pomegranates are a symbol of fertility because of their many seeds, yet of death because of the vivid blood red of the pulp. (See life-death-rebirth deity.) In mythology, Persephone was condemned to spend time in the Underworld every year because Hades tricked her into eating six pomegranate seeds while she was his prisoner. The pomegranate was a symbol of the Aegean Triple Goddess who evolved into Olympian Hera, who is represented offering the pomegranate. See also Orion (mythology).

In the development of European iconography, the pomegranate developed into the Orb that a monarch holds at coronation. Maximilian I, Holy Roman Emperor adopted it as his personal emblem; it appears in the Emperor's hand in Albrecht Dürer's posthumous portrait of him, 1519.

A pomegranate appears in the shield of Granada.

The pomegranate gave its name to the grenade from its shape, and to the garnet from its colour.

Poppy

A poppy is an annual, biennial, or perennial plant of the Family Papaveraceae, typically with showy flowers borne one per stem, native mainly to the Northern hemisphere and often grown for ornament, opium or food. 15–100 cm high, it yields a milky sap (latex) and bears large lobed or divided leaves and white, pink, orange, or red flowers, sometimes with a dark centre, with 4–6 petals around a whorl of stamens. The fruit is a capsule with pores through which the seeds are dispersed.

Population

All the members of a given species in a particular region.

Porcine

Of, relating to, or from swine (pigs) such as porcine growth hormone.

Positional Cloning

A technique used to identify genes, usually those that are associated with diseases, based on their location on a chromosome. This is contrast to the older, "functional cloning" technique that relies on some knowledge of a gene protein product. For most diseases, researchers have no such knowledge.

Positive Pressure Personnel Suit

Personnel protection equivalent to that provided by Class III (BSCs). It is a one-piece, ventilated suit worn by the laboratory worker when working with Biosafety Level 3 (BL-3) or Biosafety Level 4 (BL-4) in a "suit area" and using Class I or II Biological Safety Cabinets (BSCs). The personnel suit is maintained under positive pressure with a life-support system to prevent leakage into the suit. In this containment system, the worker is isolated from the work materials. The personnel suit area must be entered through an airlock fitted with airtight doors. A chemical shower is provided as a "dunk tank" to decontaminate the surfaces of the suit as the worker leaves the area. The exhaust air from the suit area is filtered through two HEPA filters installed in series. The entire area must be under negative pressure.

Potable

Suitable for drinking.

Potent

A substance that is "active" in relatively low doses or concentrations.

Poultice

A hot, moist mass of linseed, mustard, or soap and soil between two pieces of muslin to relieve congestion, pain, or promote absorption of inflammatory substances, or to act as a counterirritant. Poultices often contain additional medicinal plant ingredients.

Powdered extract

Powdered extracts are prepared from native extracts by diluting to the specified strengths with diluents (e.g. starch, lactose, etc.) and/or anti-caking agents (e.g. magnesium carbonate) followed by drying, usually under vacuum, to yield dry solids. These are ground into powders to yield powdered extracts or granulated to produce granular extracts.

PP (Polypropylene)

A crystalline polymer with a melting point of 330°F (165°C), and heat deflection temperature ranging from 195°F (91°C) to 240°F (116°C) which is higher than other common plastics. Its key properties are high heat resistance (for piping an upper limit of 212°F (100°C)), a specific gravity of 0.91 if unmodified (the lightest of the most common thermoplastics), stiffness, and chemical resistance with respect to handling caustics, solvents, acids, and other organic chemicals. It is not recommended for use with oxidizing type acids, detergents, low boiling hydrocarbons, alcohols, and some chlorinated organic materials. Polypropylene is a relatively inert material and contributes little in the way of contamination to pharmaceutical water.

PPB (Parts Per Billion)

Parts per billion (abbreviated ppb only in the U.S.), or micrograms per liter. One part per billion is like seeing a bottle cap on the earth's equator from an orbiting satellite.

PPF

A blood plasma fraction. Identical to NHSA (also see: NHSA, ISG) but containing no more than 15% w/w A and ß globulins. Dispensed as a 5% solution.

PPLO

Pleuropneumonia Like Organism.

PPM (Parts Per Million)

Abbreviation for parts per million, used to describe concentration in liquids or gases, e.g., 10,000 ppm is approximately equivalent to 10 g/liter or a 1% W/V solution.

PPM (Parts Per Million)

The most common measure of dissolved ionized impurities in

water. It is the same as milligrams per liter. For discussion of ppm as a measure of Total Ionized Solids see Milliequivalent.

PQ (Performance Qualification)

Documented evidence that a process or system consistently and reproducibly performs as intended and does what it purports to do. This accomplished through extended time studies or process runs with simulated products or conditions.

Precipitate

An insoluble reaction product. When a solution reaches saturation, solute will begin to come out of solution, as when water precipitates from the air as rain, or calcium carbonate precipitates out of water to form scale, the chalky white substance deposited on the inside of tea kettles.

Precursor

Plants make phytochemicals by starting with one chemical, a 'parent compound,' and changing it into another, called a 'derivative' — meaning 'derived from the parent compound.' There is a sometimes lengthy series of chemical transformations where the original molecule changes shapes, splits up, or joins with other molecules or atoms on the way to becoming the derivative. Biochemists call this chain of transformative relationships a 'pathway.' A pathway is organized by a specific group of enzymes that help change each form of the molecule into the next form 'downstream.' A molecule that is 'upstream' in this process is called a precursor of the final molecule.

Premenstrual syndrome (PMS)

A syndrome occurring several days prior to the onset of menstruation and ending a short time after menstruation begins. Common symptoms are irritability, emotional tension, anxiety, mood swings, depression, headache, breast tenderness and/or swelling, and water retention with or without oedema.

Precommission

Preparing the plant for commissioning (start-up). This includes briefly starting (bumping) all pieces of equipment, verifying their shaft rotation is correct, verifying that valves, gauges, and other inline devices are installed in the correct orientation, and performing functionality runs on all equipment and material. This also includes leak tests.

Predicate Rules

A previously published set of rules (such as GLPs, GCP, or cGMPs) that mandate what records must be maintained, the required contents of those records, whether signatures are necessary, and how long the record must be maintained.

Prefilter

A filter to trap gross particulates located upstream before a HEPA filter. The efficiency of initial prefilters is usually in the 20% to 30% range by the ASHRAE Atmospheric Dust Spot Efficiency, while intermediate prefilters usually have a collection efficiency of 80% to 90% by the same test.

Preservative

A bacteriostatic or bacteriocidal agent added to some multiple dose parenterals and most cosmetics. Examples are benzalkonium chloride (BAC), formaldehyde, and thimerosol (merthiolate).

Pressure Rating

Pressure at which a system is designed to operate, allowing for applicable safety factors.

Pressure Vessel

A closed vessel designed to operate at pressures above 15 psig (103.4 kPa).

Pretreatment

Initial water treatment steps performed prior to final processing to prolong the life of cartridges and filters and to protect downstream elements from premature failure.

Primary Air

Air circulating through HEPA filters used to produce unidirectional flow in critical zones.

Primary Containment

The first level of containment, consisting of the inside portion of that container which comes into immediate contact on its inner surface with the material being contained.

Primary Productivity

The basis of all food chains, the production at the lowest level of the food chain...usually photosynthesis.

Primer

Short preexisting polynucleotide chain to which DNA polymerase can add new deoxyribonucleotides.

Principle of Nonrepudiation

The ability to say with confident assurance that only one user entered specific data or performed specific actions on a computer system and that the particular user is identifiable. If more than one user can get into the system in such a way that the audit trail cannot specify who performed what action, the principle of nonrepudiation has been violated.

Prions

Virus-like proteinaceous infectious agents. Prions differ from viruses in that they are not known to contain either DNA or RNA..

Probe

Single stranded DNA or RNA molecules of specific base sequence, labeled either radioactively or immunologically, that are used to detect the complementary base sequence by hybridization.

Procedures

A documented description of the operations to be carried out, the precautions to be taken and measures to be applied directly or indirectly related to the manufacture of an intermediate or API.

Process Aids

Materials, excluding solvents, used as an aid in the

manufacture of an intermediate or API (Active Pharmaceutical Ingredient) which themselves do not participate in a chemical or biological reaction (e.g. filter aid, activated carbon, etc.).

Process Limits

Environmental limits that, if exceeded, may affect product quality adversely.

Process Suitability

The established capacity of the manufacturing process to produce effective and reproducible results consistently.

Process Support Systems

Systems that do not contact product and are generally engineering systems.

Process Systems

Systems that may contact the drug substance or could otherwise directly impact product quality.

Process Validation

Establishing, through documented evidence, a high degree of assurance that a specific process will consistently produce a product that meets its predetermined specifications and quality characteristics.

Process Validation Protocol

Documented plan for testing a pharmaceutical product and process to confirm that the production process used to manufacture the product performs as intended. This includes a review of process variables and operational limitations as well as providing the sampling plan under actual use conditions.

Product Campaign

The production of more than one product in a facility, with strict adherence to accepted cleaning procedures between these products. The products may be run in the same equipment, but not at the same time.

Product Contact Surface

A surface that contacts raw materials, process materials, and/or product.

Product Mix

The types and number of different products produced in a facility.

Product Water

The water produced as a result of a treatment process.

Production

All operations involved in the preparation of an API (Active Pharmaceutical Ingredient), from receipt of materials, through processing and packaging, to its completion as a finished API.

Progesterone

A steroid hormone secreted by the corpus luteum and placenta. It governs changes in the endometrium in the second half of the menstrual cycle preparatory for implantation of the blastocyst (fertilized egg cell), development of the maternal placenta after implantation, and development or mammary glands.

Prokaryote

A unicellular organism having a less complex structure than a eukaryote. It is characterized by the absence of a nucleus and by having the genetic material in the form of simple filaments of DNA. The sizes of most prokaryotes vary from 0.5μm to 3μm in equivalent radius. Different species have different shapes such as spherical or Coccus (for example, Staphylococci), cylindrical or bacillus (E. coli), or spiral or spirillum (Rhodospirillum).

Promoter

A site on DNA to which RNA polymerase will bind and initiate transcription.

Pro-oxidant

Opposite of an antioxidant; causes oxidation.

Prophylactic Surgery

Surgery to remove tissue that is in danger of becoming cancerous, before cancer has the chance to develop. Surgery to remove the breasts of women at high risk of developing breast cancer is known as prophylactic mastectomy.

Prophylaxis

The prevention of, or protective treatment for disease.

Propylene Glycol

A common solvent for antibiotics, particularly the tetracyclines. Miscible (soluble) in water, but often filtered as pure propylene glycol prior to combination with the antibiotic. Its high viscosity controls absorption of the dissolved drug.

Prospective Validation

Establishing documented evidence that a system does what it purports to do based on a preplanned protocol.

Prostaglandins

A large group of biologically active, 20-carbon, unsaturated fatty acids that represent various metabolites or arachidonic acid. They are local, short-range autacoids, which exert their effects locally and then are destroyed enzymatically. They influence or control a wide variety or physiological functions, including fluid balance, platelet aggregation, gastrointestinal activity, neurotransmission, endocrine functions, etc.

Prosthetic Groups

Organic and/or inorganic components other than amino acids, contained in proteins.

Prostrate

A gland that surrounds the neck of the bladder and the urethra in the male. It secretes an alkaline fluid that is part of the seminal fluid.

Prostrate-specific antigen (PSA)

A marker for cancer of the prostrate found in the bloodstream, excreted by both benign tumors, e.g., those found in BPH, and malignant tumors, but from malignant tumors at much higher concentrations.

Protease

A proteolytic enzyme; a protein that can cleave other proteins into smaller fragments.

Protein

One of a group of substances constituting the greater part of the nitrogen-containing components of animal and vegetable tissues. They are of very complex constitution, all containing carbon, hydrogen, nitrogen, and oxygen and some containing in addition iron, phosphorous, or sulfur; chemically they are regarded as peptides (polypeptides) or combinations of amino acids and their derivatives. They are colorless, odorless, generally tasteless, and of varying degrees of solubility; they are putrefiable and readily undergo chemical change, hydrolysis, under the influence of ferments and on boiling with dilute acids or alkalis.

Protein Sequencer

An instrument that will determine the sequence of amino acids, which make up a particular protein.

Proteolysis

Protein hydrolysis, the decomposition of protein.

Proteolytic Enzyme (Protease)

Any enzyme that takes part in the breaking down of proteins. A system of several such enzymes is necessary to break down proteins to their constituent amino acids.

Proteomics

A concept more than a defined technology, it refers to any protein-based approach that has the capacity to provide new information about proteins on a genomewide scale. 75% of the predicted proteins in multicellular organisms have no known cellular function.

Protocol

A prospective plan, that when executed as intended, produces documented evidence that a Process or System has been properly qualified.

Protoplasm

A semifluid, viscous, translucent mixture of water, proteins, lipids, carbohydrates, and inorganic salts found in all plant and animal cells.

Protozoa

Nucleated microorganisms, some of which are large enough to be detected with the naked eye. They consist of a single cell and or an aggregation of nondifferentiated cells loosely held together and not forming tissues. The protozoa are divided into four classes: Sarcodina, Mastigophora, Sporozoa, and Infusoria (Ciliata).

PRP

Pressure-x-rate product. A measurement of cardiac capacity, frequently measured on an ergometric bicycle. A lower number (multiplicative product) indicates better capacity.

Pseudonomas Diminuta

The bacterium used for validation of sterilizing filters. Recognized as the challenge organism for 0.2µm filters, its size is 0.3 x 0.8µm approximately. According to the HIMA (Health Industries Manufacturers Association) standard, filters must be successfully challenged to a titre of 107 per cm^2 to be validated as sterilizing grade 0.2µm rated.

Psychrophile

An organism that requires temperatures below 20°C (68°F) for growth.

Psychrometer

A hygrometer that uses the difference in readings between two thermometers, one having a wet bulb ventilated to cause evaporation and the other having a dry bulb, as a measure of atmospheric moisture.

Psychrometry

Determination of the properties of gas-vapor mixtures. The air-water vapor system is by far the one most commonly encountered.

Psychosomatic

Pertaining to the relationship between the mind and the body.

PTFE (Polytetrafluoroethylene) Teflon®

A fluoroplastic that is resistant to practically every known chemical or solvent in combination with the highest useful temperature limit of commercially available plastics. PTFE has a melt point of 620°F (327°C), a useful temperature range from -436°F (-260°C) to 500°F (260°C), high impact strength, and exceptionally low coefficient of friction. Usual processing techniques like injection molding are not possible with PTFE due to a very high molecular weight which results in a melt viscosity about 1 million times higher than is acceptable for conventional thermoplastics. PTFE resin is pressed into shapes under high pressure at room temperature and then heated to 700°F (371°C) to complete the molding (sintering process) and adjust the crystalline content.

Public Key Certificate (PKC)

A data file issued by a certified authority to a person or company that acquires a digital signature service. The certificate includes information identifying the subject, the issuing authority, and the period of validity, and it provides the related public key. The certified authority signs the PKC digitally.

Pure Culture

A culture containing only one species of microorganism.

Pure Steam

Steam that is produced by a steam generator which, when condensed, meets requirements for WFI.

Punarnava

Punarnava consists of the fresh or the dried plant, *Boerhaavia diffusa* Linn.

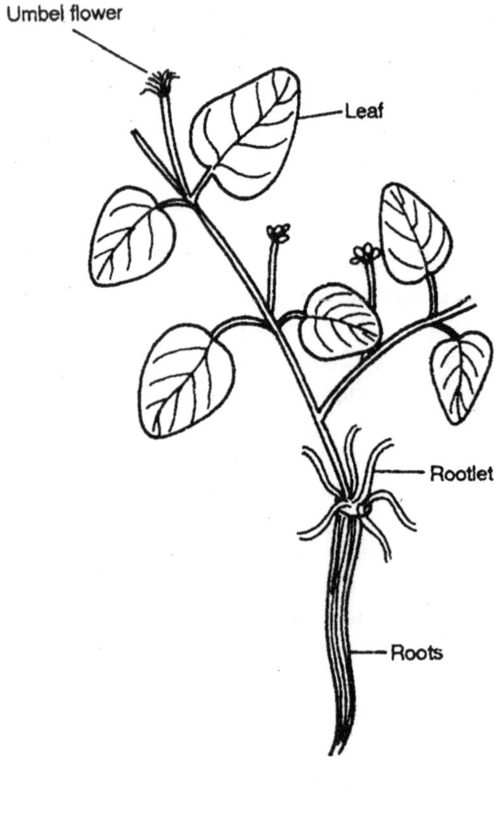

Punarnava

Purification

The removal of impurities of concern. The term has one meaning when applied to the preparation of drinking water, another when applied to reagent grade water for the laboratory, and still another when applied to water used to rinse ICs (Integrated Circuit devices).

Purified Water, U.S.P.

Water rendered suitable for pharmaceutical purposes by

processes such as distillation, ion-exchange treatment (deionization or demineralization), or reverse osmosis. It meets rigid specifications for chemical purity, the requirements of the Federal Environmental Protection Agency (EPA) with respect to drinking water, and it contains no added substances. Cannot be used as raw material for parenterals. Common uses are: a rinse for equipment, vials, and ampoules, and as make up for cosmetics, bulk chemicals, and oral products. For FDA acceptance, purified water must contain less than 0.5 mg/l of TOC (Total Organic Carbon), and less than 100 CFU (Colony Forming Units).

Purine

A nitrogen-containing, double-ring, basic compound that occurs in nucleic acids. The purines in DNA and RNA are adenine and guanine.

Purity

The ratio of desirable to undesirable components in a liquid as determined on a weight basis per unit volume of sample.

PVC (Polyvinyl Chloride)

The largest volume of the vinyl family of plastics. Overall it has excellent basic properties, may be easily processed and welded, and is exceptionally economical in cost. Homopolymers grades of PVC comprise over 80% of all PVC used, and contain 56.8% chlorine by weight. When the chlorine content is increased to about 67% its heat deflection temperature at 264 psi increases from 155°F (68°C) to 218°F (103°C). Because PVC is a thermally sensitive thermoplastic compounding ingredients such as heat stabilizers, lubricants, fillers, plasticizers, impact modifiers, pigments, and processing aids must be added to make it processible. PVC is prone to produce extractables during start-up in high purity water.

PVDF (Polyvinylidene Fluoride)

A thermoplastic fluoropolymer with a melt point of 352°F (178°C), and a wide service range from -40°F (-40°C) to 284°F (140°C). It has a very linear chemical structure, and is similar to PTFE with the exception of not being fully fluorinated, i.e. having 3% hydrogen by weight. Its drawbacks in the area of chemical resistance include unsuitability with strong alkalis, fuming acids, polar solvents, amines, ketones, and esters. It has a high tensile strength as well as a high heat deflection temperature. It is readily weldable, offers high purity qualities, and is resistant to permeation of gases. PVDF is a relatively inert material and contributes little in the way of contamination to pharmaceutical water.

Pyrethrum

Pyrethrum consists of the dried, closed or half open flowers of *Chrysanthemum* cinerarifolium Vis.

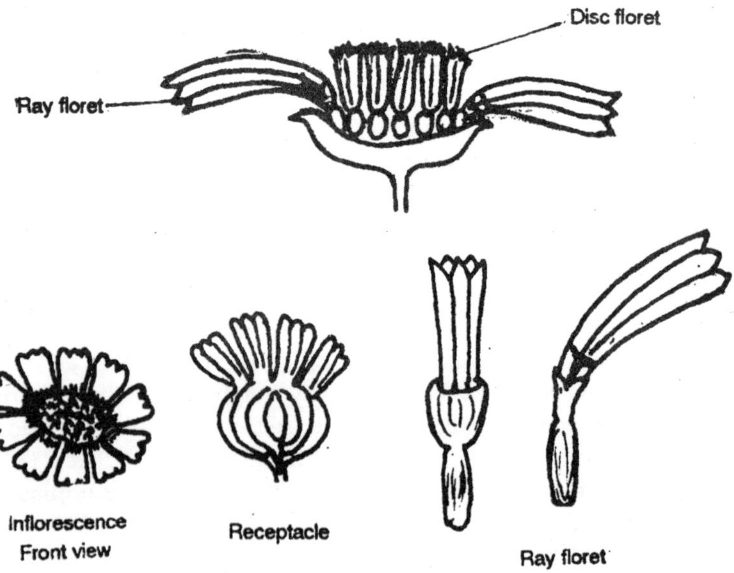

Pyrethrum

Pyridoxine

One of a group of substances, including pyridoxal and pyridoxamine that make up vitamin B6.

Pyrimidine

A nitrogen-containing, single ring, basic compound that occurs in nucleic acids. The pyrimidines in DNA are cytosine and thymine, in RNA, cytosine, and uracil. (also see: Purine) Pyrogen A foreign substance that produces a fever response in humans and animals, hence the name pyrogen (heat producing). Chemically, the lipopolysaccharide outer layer of gram-negative bacteria. Bacterial pyrogens were at one time believed to be toxic substances released when bacterial cells disintegrate and are therefore still referred to as endotoxins. Parenteral drugs must be essentially pyrogen free. (also see; Lipopolysaccharide (LPS), Endotoxin) Pyrophoric A chemical that will spontaneously ignite in air at or below a temperature of 130°F (54.5°C).

Q

QA (Quality Assurance)

The sum total of the organized arrangements made to ensure that all APIs (Active Pharmaceutical Ingredients) are of the quality required for their intended use and that quality systems are maintained.

QC (Quality Control)

Checking or testing, that specifications are met, or the regulatory process through which the industry measures actual quality performance, compares it with standards, and acts on the difference.

Qualification

Action of providing that equipment or ancillary systems are properly installed, work correctly, and actually lead to the expected results. Qualification is part of validation, but the individual qualification steps alone do not constitute process validation.

Quality Assurance (QA) Group

The group who interprets the GMP regulations and guidelines.

Quality Control (QC) Group

The group who enforces the GMP regulations.

Quality Unit(s)

An organizational unit independent of production that fulfills both Quality Assurance and Quality Control responsibilities. This may be in the form of separate QA and QC units, a single individual (or group), depending upon the size and structure of the organization.

Quality Function

The entire collection of activities from which the industry achieves fitness for use, no matter where these activities are performed.

Quarantine

The status of materials isolated physically or by other effective means pending a decision on their subsequent approval or rejection.

Queen of the Meadow Root (Eupatorum purpureum)

Also known as gravel root or Joe-Pye Weed. Diuretic, anti-lithic, urinary infections, respiratory.

Quick Stop

DNA mutants of E. coli cease replication immediately when the temperature is increased to 42°C.

R

R

In molecular structure, 'R' is a kind of shorthand that stands for a variable group; for example, in a set of related molecules that are mostly identical, you might find $-CH_3$ attached to a particular spot in one molecule, $-C_3H_5$ in the corresponding place in the second molecule, and simply -H in that spot in the third molecule. R is a way of saying, 'this could be any one of a number of structures.'

Radiation Sterilization

Sterilization using gamma radiation emitted from radioactive materials such as cobalt-60, or cesium 137. If proper dosage of nuclear radiation can be documented, sterility testing is not required.

Radio-Immunoassay (RIA)

A highly sensitive method of detecting and measuring the concentration of biological compounds in vivo.

Radioactive Material

A material or combination of materials that spontaneously emits ionizing radiation.

Random controlled trial

An experimental procedure for assessing the effects of a

particular variable (such as a drug) in which patients are assigned on a random basis to either of two groups, experimental or control. The experimental groups receive the drug or treatment, while the control group does not.

Randomisation

In research studies, a method used to assign subjects to experimental groups. Helps to prevent inadvertent selection bias in the study.

Raw Material

A general term used to denote starting materials, reagents, intermediates, process aids, and solvents intended for use in the production of intermediates or APIs (Active Pharmaceutical Ingredients).

rDNA (Recombinant DNA)

The hybrid DNA produced by joining pieces of DNA from different sources.

Reactive oxygen species (ROS)

Damaging molecules, including oxygen radicals (i.e. superoxide radical) and other highly reactive forms of oxygen (i.e. singlet oxygen) that can harm biomolecules and contribute to disease states. Other oxygen-containing radicals, such as the hydroxyl and peroxyl radicals, are often classified as ROS too.

Reagent

A substance used (as in detecting or measuring a component, in preparing a product, or in developing photographs) because of its chemical or biological activity.

Reagent Grade Water

Water suitable for use in making up reagents or for use in sensitive analytical procedures. There are several grades of reagent grade water as defined by various professional organizations, such as ASTM, CAP, NCCLS, and ACS:

1. Type I: Used for procedures requiring maximum accuracy and precision, such as atomic spectrometry, flame photometry,

enzymology, blood gas, pH and specific ion determinations; reference buffer solutions; and reconstitution of lyophilized materials used as standards. ASTM to produce Type I water specifies distillation pretreatment of feedwater.
2. Type II: Recommended for most analytical or general laboratory testing such as hematological, seralogical, and microbiological procedures as well as chemical methods not specifically stated or proven to require Type I quality. ASTM specifies preparation of Type II by distillation and recommends it whenever freedom from organic impurities is important.
3. Type III: Satisfactory for some general laboratory tests; for most qualitative analyses such as urinalysis, parasitology, and histological procedures; for rinsing of analytical samples; preparation of stock solutions; and for washing or rinsing of glassware (final glassware rinsing should be performed with the water type specified for the procedure performed). Distillation, mixed-bed deionization, and reverse osmosis (with high quality feedwater) can be used to generate Type III.

Recalcification

A technique producing serum from anticoagulated plasma. Citrate and oxalate act as anticoagulants because they are Ca++ (Calcium Ion) chelating agents; Ca++ as calcium chloride is added in excess (1/40 Molar). Ca++ is a coagulation co-factor (catalyst) and promotes clot formation.

Recalcitrant Molecules

Molecules which are not readily degraded under normal environmental conditions.

Recessive Allele

A gene that is expressed only when its counterpart allele on the matching chromosome is also recessive (not dominant). Autosomal recessive disorders develop in persons who receive two copies of the mutant gene, one from each parent who is a carrier.

Recirculation

Continuous recirculation may be necessary to maintain uniformly high purity in larger water systems. Water is continuously recirculated and reprocessed to prevent stagnation and to rinse out residual impurities in the system. Bacteria flourish in stagnant water, especially if temperature is conducive to growth.

Recombinant

Pertaining to the recombining of generic material from one species into alternate sequences. Plasmids may then be used to incorporate the genetic material into other organisms such as E. coli bacteria.

Recombinant Clone

Clone containing recombinant DNA molecules.

Recombinant DNA Molecules

In the context of the NIH Guidelines, recombinant DNA molecules are those constructed outside living cells by joining natural or synthetic DNA segments to DNA molecules that can replicate in a living cell, or molecules that result from the replication of those described above.

Recombinant DNA (rDNA)

The hybrid DNA produced by joining pieces of DNA from different sources.

Recombinant DNA Techniques

Procedures that transfer genetic material between organisms or species.

Recombinant DNA Technology

Procedure used to join together DNA segments in a cell-free system (an environment outside a cell or organism). Under appropriate conditions, a recombinant DNA molecule can enter a cell and replicate there, either autonomously or after it has become integrated into a cellular chromosome.

Recombination

The process by which progeny derive a combination of genes different from that of either parent. In higher organisms, this can occur by crossing over.

Recovery

Any treatment of materials by a process intended to make them suitable for further use.

Recovery Time

The time after an upset in a room's HVAC environmental parameters for the room to return to "normal" conditions, such as a return to acceptable humidity levels after a room wash down. This occurs within a certain number of air changes after the upset source is removed, minimally six to ten, depending on the severity of the upset, the quality of the air supply, and the degree of mixing of room air.

Red raspberry leaves (Rubus idaeus)

A uterine tonic59; relaxes the uterus; traditionally believed to lead to an easier childbirth60; midwives have found that women who drink raspberry leaf tea regularly during pregnancy have decreased chance of hemorrhage; relieves kidney irritation61.

Red clover (Trifolium pratense)

Helps treat gout; reduces coughing62; expels mucous from the lungs and throat; used to treat and prevent cancer.

Red root (Ceanothus americanus)

Treats tonsil inflammations and sore throats; increases transport of nutrients from the blood across the capillary cells to the lymph.

Reference Standard, Primary

A substance that has been shown by an extensive set of analytical tests, to be authentic material of high purity. This standard may be obtained from a recognized source or may be prepared by independent synthesis or by further purification of existing production material.

Reference Standard, Secondary A substance of established quality and purity, as shown by comparison to a primary reference standard, used as a reference standard for routine laboratory analysis.

Referential Integrity

Relationship between records that ensures data integrity by maintaining unbreakable links between related electronic records. It ensures confidence that a specific record (such as a calculated chromatographic result) is unmodified, unmanipulated, and otherwise uncorrupted after its creation and that still carries the references to the other electronic records that were used to generate it.

Refrigerants

Fluids used for heat transfer in a refrigerating system; the refrigerant absorbs heat and transfers it at a higher temperature and higher pressure, usually with a change of state. Refrigerants can be: 1. Primary refrigerants. Liquids with low boiling points that change from a liquid to a gas after absorbing heat. 2. Secondary refrigerants. Substances that act only as heat carriers, such as brine, air, and water.

Regenerate

Restore ion exchange of resins by reversing the process. An acid rinse is used to restore cation resin capacity and a sodium hydroxide rinse is used to restore anion resin capacity.

Regulatory Affairs

Drug companies must show that their products consistently meet standards set by government agencies. Regulatory affairs departments document those activities, submit proposals, and follow those proposals through completion or approval.

Regulatory Region or Sequence

A DNA base sequence that controls gene expression.

Reishi Mushroom (Ganoderma sinensis)

An immunostimulant.

Reject Stream

In reverse osmosis and ultrafiltration, those impurities not able to permeate the membrane are said to be rejected (removed). They are flushed away in the reject (waste) stream.

Relational Database Management System (RDBMS)

A type of database system that stores data in related tables. A relational database is powerful because it does not assume how data are related or how they will be extracted from the database. As a result, the same database can be viewed in many different ways.

Relative Humidity (% RH)

The ratio (measured in percent) of actual water vapor pressure in air to the pressure of saturated water vapor in air at the same temperature and pressure.

Release

The discharge of a microbiological agent or eukaryotic cell from a containment system.

Renaturation

The restoration of biological activity to a denatured protein or nucleic acid. The strands of a DNA duplex, for example, are denatured at high temperatures but can be correctly reformed by a slow cooling.

Representative Sample

A sample that consists of a number of units that are drawn based on rational criteria such as random sampling and intended to assure that the sample accurately portraits the material being sampled.

Reprocessing

A system of reworking batches that do not conform to standards or specifications, including "the steps taken to ensure that the reprocessed batches will conform to all established standards, specifications, and characteristics".

Reprocessing (ICH API definition)

Introducing an intermediate or API, including that which does not conform to standards or specifications, back into the process and repeating a crystallization step or other appropriate chemical or physical manipulation steps (e.g., distillation, filtration, chromatography, milling, etc.) that are part of the established manufacturing process. Continuation of a chemical reaction after an in-process control test shows the reaction to be incomplete is considered to be part of the normal process, and not reprocessing.

Reproductive Toxicology

Studies of whether exposure affects male or female fertility.

Resin

An amorphous exudate of certain plants, typically consisting of polysaccharides and oxidised terpenes.

2. Ion exchange resins are usually bead-like spherical materials with an affinity for particular ions. Cation exchange resins made of styrene and divinylbenzene containing sulfonic acid groups will exchange hydrogen ions for any cations they encounter. Similarly, anion exchange resins made of styrene and divinylbenzene containing quaternary ammonium groups will exchange a hydroxyl ion for any anions.

Resistance (Filter)

The pressure drop across a filter at a stated flow and under given conditions; generally expressed in millimeters water gauge or PSI, or in SI units as N/m^2 or Pascals.

Resistivity The reciprocal of conductivity (R=1/C). A measure of specific resistance to the flow of electricity. In water, provides an easy mean of continuously measuring the purity of very low Total Dissolved Solids (TDS), or ionic concentration. The fewer the dissolved ions in water, the higher its resistivity. Resistivity is normally expressed in Megohm-cm and is equivalent to one million ohms of resistance measured between two electrodes one centimeter apart. The theoretical maximum ionic purity of water is 18.3 Megohm-cm at 25°C.

Resolution

Degree of molecular detail on a physical map of DNA, ranging from low to high.

Restriction Enzyme, Endonuclease

A protein that recognizes specific, short nucleotide sequences and cuts DNA at those sites. Bacteria contain over 400 such enzymes that recognize and cut over 100 different DNA sequences.

Restriction Enzyme Cutting Site

A specific nucleotide sequence of DNA at which a particular restriction enzyme cuts the DNA. Some sites occur frequently in DNA (e.g., every several hundred base pairs), others much less frequently (rarecutter; e.g., every 10,000 base pairs).

Restriction Fragment Length Polymorphism (RFLP)

Variation between individuals in DNA fragments sizes cut by specific restriction enzymes; polymorphic sequences that result in RFLPs are used as markers on both physical maps and genetic linkage maps. RFLPs are usually caused by mutation at a cutting site.

Retest Date

The date when samples of the API (Active Pharmaceutical Ingredient)a material should be re-examined to ensure that material is still suitable for use.

Retinoblastoma

An eye cancer caused by the loss of a pair of tumor-suppressor genes; the inherited form typically appears in childhood, since one gene is missing from the time of birth.

Retrospective Validation

Establishing documented evidence that a system does what it purports to do based on review and analysis of historic information.

Retrovirus

An oncogenic, RNA-containing virus, which replicates through a double-stranded DNA intermediate necessitating the presence of an RNA-dependent DNA polymerase.

Revalidation

Repetition of validation process or a specific portion of it.

Revalidation

Extent of validation necessary to assure that changes made to qualified or validated equipment, utilities, systems and process do not adversely affect the finished product. Implemented changes should be tracked and evaluated through a thorough, dynamic, change control program.

Reverse Osmosis (RO)

The reversal of osmosis to purify water. In osmosis, water diffuses through a semipermeable membrane from a region of higher concentration (such as pure fresh water) into one of lower concentration (such as a solution of water and salt). The flow of water can be reversed with an opposing pressure that exceeds osmotic pressure. With RO, water is forced out of the lower concentrated solution (such as the salt solution), leaving the solute (impurities) behind.

Reverse Osmosis (RO)

RO is one of two acceptable techniques for producing Water For injection (WFI), U.S.P. Procedure involves passing purified water across a semipermeable membrane against an osmotic gradient. R.O. is an excellent pretreatment for deionized water that will be subsequently filtered, because silt and colloids are removed. Usual performance of R.O. is removal of organics, multi-valent ions, and 90% of mono-valent ions.

Reworking

Subjecting an intermediate or API (Active Pharmaceutical Ingredient) that does not conform to standards or specifications, to one or more processing steps that are different from the established manufacturing process so that its quality may be made acceptable (e.g., recrystallizing with a different solvent).

Rhubarb root (Rheum palmateom)

The root stimulates the appetite; helps stop diarrhea; inhibits bacterial growth63; inhibits growth of cancer64; sometimes administered for upper digestive tract bleeding65.

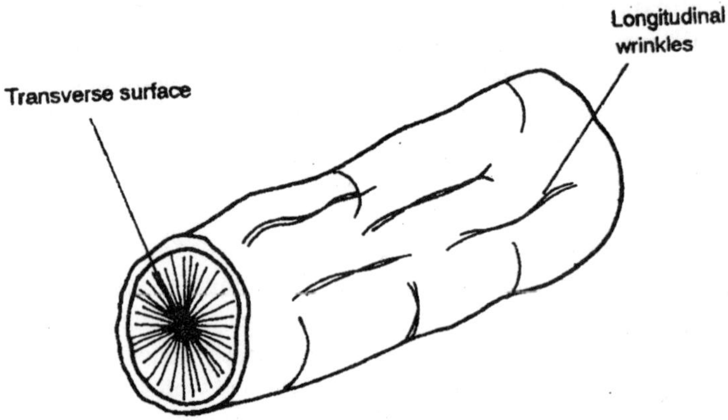

Rhubarb

Ribosomes

Small cellular components composed of specialized ribosomal RNA and protein; site of protein synthesis.

Rickettsias

Gram-negative microorganisms that are often carried by arthropod vectors and may infect humans and other mammals. Generally smaller than other bacteria, they require living cells for growth.

Rinse

The operation that follows regeneration, a flushing out of excess regenerant solution.

Roller Bottles

Small cylindrical bottles often used as bioreactors in the production of products by cell culture. The bottles are kept on a device that rotates them slowly to help assure proper growth. Automated systems may also be used for large arrays of roller bottles int oducing sterile media and harvesting finished product automatically.

Rosemary (Rosemarinus officinalis)

Treats headaches; soothes upset stomach; a muscle stimulant; soothes irritated nerves66.

Rouge

Form of surface corrosion that occurs in some stainless steel piping systems.

Roughness

Consists of the finer irregularities of the surface texture, usually including those irregularities that result from the manufacturing process. These are considered to include traverse feed marks and other irregularities within the limits of the roughness sampling length.

S

Saccharomyces Cerevisiae

Better known as beer yeast, ordinary yeast. Yeast used in rDNA research.

Safflower

Safflower is a highly branched, herbaceous, thistle-like annual, usually with many long sharp spines on the leaves. Plants are 30 to 150 cm tall with globular flower heads (capitula) and commonly, brilliant yellow, orange or red flowers which bloom in July. Each branch will usually have from one to five flower heads containing 15 to 20 seeds per head. Safflower has a strong taproot which enables it to thrive in dry climates, but the plant is very susceptible to frost injury from stem elongation to maturity.

Traditionally, the crop was grown for its flowers, used for colouring and flavouring foods and making red and yellow dyes, especially before cheaper aniline dyes became available, and in medicines. For the last fifty years or so, the plant has been cultivated mainly for the vegetable oil extracted from its seeds, which was formerly used in the paint industry. Today, it is used mainly as cooking oil, salad oil and for the production of margarine.

There are two types of safflower that produce different kinds of oil: one high in monounsaturated fatty acid (oleic acid) and the other high in polyunsaturated fatty acid (linoleic acid). Currently the predominant oil market is for the former, which is lower in saturates and higher in monounsaturates than olive oil, for example.

Safflower is one of humanity's oldest crops, but is a minor crop today, with about 600 000 t being produced commercially in more than sixty countries worldwide. India, United States, and Mexico are the leading producers, with Ethiopia, Kazakhstan, China, Argentina and Australia accounting for most of the remainder.

Safflower flowers are occasionally used as a cheaper substitute for saffron. Safflower seed is also used quite commonly as an alternative to sunflower seed in birdfeeders, as squirrels do not like the taste of it.

Saffron

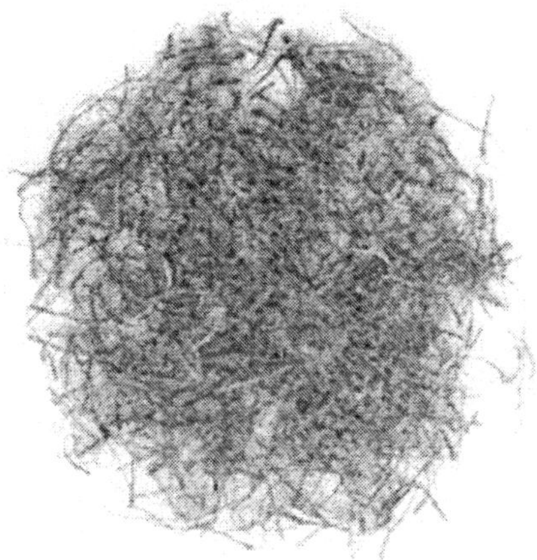

Saffron is the name given to the dried stigmata and part of the style of the saffron crocus, traditionally called Crocus sativus, which are harvested, dried, and used for cooking. Saffron has a pleasant spicy smell, and it contains a dye that colors food a distinctive deep golden colour. Safflower, Carthamus tinctorius, is often used as a less expensive substitute for saffron, as is turmeric, Curcuma longa, which mimics saffron's color well but has a very different flavour.

In European cuisine, saffron is, for example, used in many Spanish recipes, including paella and Fabada Asturiana, and in the most famous saffron-based Italian dish, the risotto alla milanese. Outside Europe, it is a vital ingredient of many Indian, Arabian and Central Asian dishes. In herbal medicine, saffron is used for its eupeptic, carminative, and emmenagogic properties.

The saffron crocus is a natural chromosome mutation, a sterile triploid variant of an eastern Mediterranean autumn-flowering crocus, C. cartwrightianus, that may have originated in Crete. Being sterile, the plant must be propagated by human aid, lifting and dividing the corms.

Saffron stigma found in Sumerian sites provide evidence that saffron was an article of long-distance trade before the Minoan palace-culture reached a peak in the 2nd millennium BC. Written records show that saffron has been used medicinally in the treatment of 90 illnesses for over four millennia. According to recent research based on Minoan frescoes on the island of Santorini in the Aegean, saffron may have been used as a medicine in the 15th century BC. Persian Saffron (Crocus sativus var. Hausknechtii) was cultivated at Derbena and Isfahan in Iran in the 10th Century.

The word "saffron" in English is also used for a shade of yellow as well as to refer to the plant. Though it is the most expensive spice in the world, saffron has also been used as a fabric dye. Traditionally, clothes colored by this particularly luminous dye were worn by the noble classes, giving the plant a ritualized caste significance.

Spain, India, and Iran are producers of saffron. Saffron is expensive because of the difficulty of extracting the stigmata of the crocus individually by hand and the number of croci it takes to make up a given weight, because the aromatic parts are so small. A pound (1/2 kg) of saffron requires approximately 35,000 - 100,000 flowers - depending on the size of each stigma; each crocus contributes three.

In England during the 15th-18th centuries, saffron was grown extensively in parts of Cambridgeshire and Essex. The Essex town of Saffron Walden got its name as a market center for the saffron trade.

Safranin

A base, obtained from aniline; aniline pink; used as a stain in histology.

Saint John's Wort (Hypericum perforatum)

Anti-inflammatory; treats lung diseases; urinary infections; helps reduce stress; helps heal wounds and cuts.

Salinity

The concentration of soluble minerals (mainly salts of the alkali metals or of magnesium) in water.

Salmonella

A large genus of the tribe Salmonellae, family Enterobacteriaceae, containing motile, gram-negative, rod-shaped organisms that ferment dextrose, forming acid and usually gas. Several species occur as intestinal pathogens in acute inflammations in humans and domestic animals. Salmonella typhimurium causes food poisoning in humans.

Salt

A compound formed by the interaction of an acid and a base, the hydrogen atoms of the acid being replaced by another positive ion derived from the base.

Salt Rejection

In reverse osmosis, the ratio of salts removed (rejected) to the original salt concentration.

"Salvage" Plasma

Plasma obtained by centrifugation of outdated (older than 21 days) whole blood. This type of plasma is difficult to convert to serum because most coagulation factors have lost their activity.

Sanitization

That part of decontamination that reduces viable microorganisms to a defined acceptance level, normally achieved by using a chemical agent or heat.

Saponins

Glycosides found in some plants, which form a lather in aqueous solutions, and cause the hemolysis of red blood cells even in high dilutions.

Saponification

Alkaline hydrolysis of triacyl glycerols to yield fatty acids as soaps.

Sarcoma

A type of cancer that starts in bone or muscle.

Sarsaparilla (Smilax ornata)

Root used to soothe sore eyes, wounds, and burns; antimicrobial as a result of antibiotic properties (saponins)67; diuretic; diaphoretic.

Saturated Air

When there is a state of mutual equilibrium between the moist air and the liquid or solid phases of water. Saturated air holds as much water vapor as it can for a given temperature and pressure.

Saturated fat

Term applied to a lipid compound with the maximum number of hydrogen atoms, where there are no double or triple bonds between the carbon atoms.

Saturated Fatty Acids

Fatty acids containing fully saturated alkyl chains.

Saturation Humidity

The air is saturated when the partial pressure of water vapor in the air at a given temperature equals the vapor pressure of water at the same temperature.

Saturation Index

The relation of calcium carbonate to the pH, alkalinity, and hardness of water to determine its scale-forming tendency.

Saw Palmetto (Serenoa serrulata)

Anti-inflammatory; appetite stimulant; digestive aid; diuretic; relives dysmenorrhea that results from lack of uterine tone.

Scale

The mineral deposit that can coat the insides of boilers or the surfaces of RO membranes. It consists mainly of calcium carbonate that precipitates out of solution under certain conditions of pH, alkalinity, and hardness.

Scale-up

To take a biopharmaceutical manufacturing process from the laboratory scale to a scale at which it is commercially feasible.

Scratch

An elongated mar in the metal's surface not associated with the predominant surface texture pattern, which is visible to the unaided eye.

Scullcap (Scutellaria lateriflora)

Nervine; relaxant68; sleep-inducing, relieves pain caused by spasms69.

Scurvy

A nutritional deficiency disease characterised by hemorrhagic manifestations and abnormal formation of bones and teeth; results from a deficiency of vitamin C.

Secondary Containment

Level of containment that is external to and separate from primary containment.

Secure Retention

The ability to generate accurate and complete copies of records in both human-readable and electronic form suitable for inspection, review, and copying by FDA. Records must be protected to enable their accurate and ready retrieval through the records retention period.

Seed Lot

Seed Lot System - A seed lot system is a system according to which successive batches of a product are derived from the same master seed lot at a given passage level. For routine production, a working seed lot is prepared from the master seed lot. The final product is derived from the working seed lot and has not undergone more passages from the master seed lot than the vaccine shown in clinical studies to be satisfactory with respect to safety and efficacy. The origin and the passage history of the master seed lot and the working seed lot are recorded.

Master Seed Lot - A culture of a microorganism distributed from a single bulk into containers in a single operation in such a manner as to ensure uniformity, to prevent contamination and to ensure stability. A master seed lot in liquid form is usually stored at or below -70°C. A freeze-dried master seed lot is stored at a temperature known to ensure stability.

Working Seed Lot - A culture of microorganism derived from the master seed lot and intended for use in production. Working seed lots are distributed into containers and stored as described above for master seed lots.

Seed Stock

The initial inoculum, or the cells placed in growth medium from which other cells will grow.

Seed Tank Industrial fermentations are generally started in tanks smaller than a 1,000 to 50,000 gallon main fermenter. This small "seed" tank may be up to 100 gallons and propagate enough organisms to "kick-off" the main fermentation. Often, a seed tank may be large enough to require its own seed tank.

Sedimentation

A primary step in municipal water treatment. Water is allowed to stand long enough for solids to settle by gravity. Also called settling.

Segregated

Storage in the same room or inside area, but physically separated by distance from incompatible materials.

Self Draining

Capable of elimination of all fluid from the system due to the force of gravity alone.

SEM (Scanning Electron Microscopy)

Utilizes an electron beam to produce images over a very broad magnification range of 10X to 105X. The technique is somewhat limited by the conductivity of the material but works very well to inspect 316L stainless steel. Typical magnification levels for surface defect evaluation are from 100 to 4,000.

Semipermeable

Membranes that do not have measurable pores but through which smaller molecules can pass.

Semiautomatic Arc Welding

Arc welding with equipment that controls only the filler metal feed. The advance of the welding is manually controlled.

Senna

The drug consists of dried leaflets and pods of *Cassia angustifolia* Vahl (Tinnevelly senna) or *Cassia acutifolia* Delile (Alexendrian senna).

Sensible Heat (SH)

Heat that causes a change of temperature without causing a change of state.

Sensible Heat Ratio

The ratio of room sensible heat to room total heat as expressed in the formula: Sensible Heat ratio (SHR) = Room Sensible Heat (SH)/Room Total Heat (TH).

Sensitizer

A chemical that causes a substantial proportion of exposed people or animals to develop an allergic reaction in normal tissue after repeated exposure to the chemical.

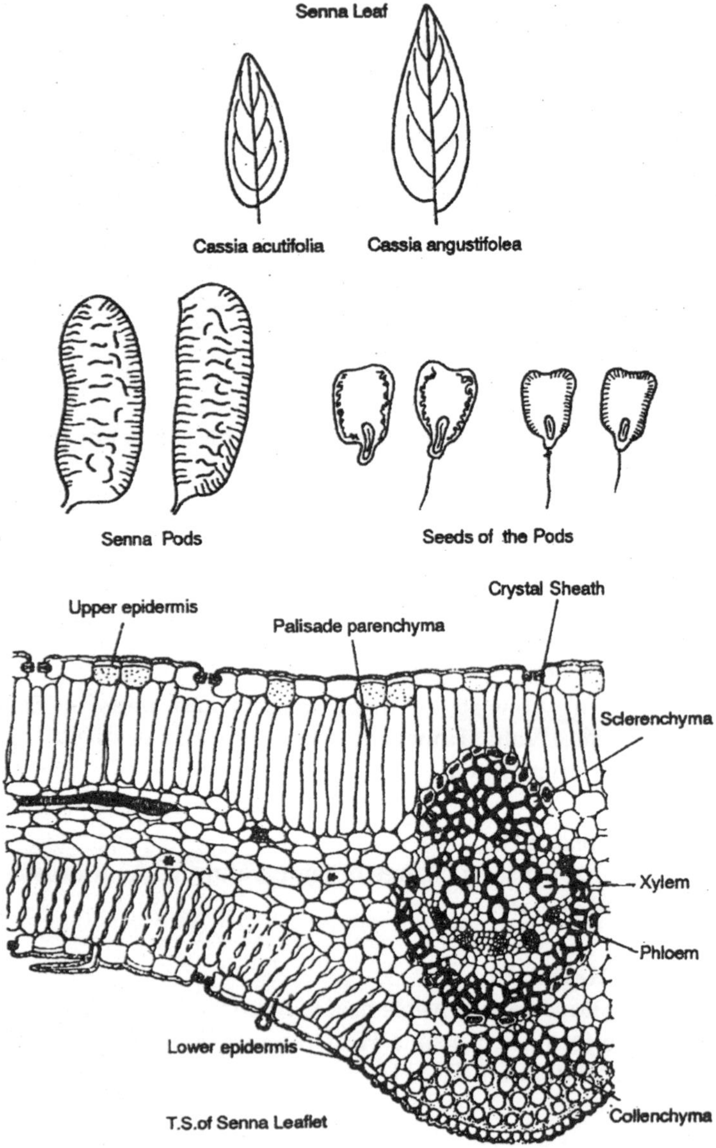
Senna Leaf
Cassia acutifolia
Cassia angustifolea
Senna Pods
Seeds of the Pods
Upper epidermis
Palisade parenchyma
Crystal Sheath
Sclerenchyma
Xylem
Phloem
Lower epidermis
Collenchyma
T.S.of Senna Leaflet

senna

Sepsis

The presence of various pus-forming and other pathogenic organisms or their toxins in the blood or tissues; septicemia.

Sequence Tagged Site (STS)

Short (200 to 500 base pairs) DNA sequence that has a single occurrence in the human genome and whose location and base sequence are known. Detectable by polymerase chain reaction, STSs are useful for localizing and orienting the mapping and sequence data reported from many different laboratories and serve as landmarks on the developing physical map of the human genome. Expressed sequence tags (ESTs) are STSs derived from cDNAs.

Sequencing (of DNA or RNA) Determination of the order of nucleotides (base sequences) in a DNA or RNA molecule or the order of amino acids in a protein.

Sera

One of the plural forms of serum.

Serratia Marcescens

They are minute, rod-shaped or coccoid, aerobic, gram-negative organisms, found on various foodstuffs as a pink or reddish growth, nonpathogenic. Used to validate 0.45μm removal rated filters.

Serotonin

5-hydroxytrptamine (5-HT), wide spread in the body, that functions as a vasoconstrictive hormone and neurotransmitter.

Serum

The water portion of the blood after coagulation, formed when coagulated blood is left standing long enough for the clot to shrink.

2. The liquid portion remaining after clotting whole blood or plasma.

Shankhpushpi

The drug consists of whole dried herb of *Convolvulus pluricaculis* and *Evolvulus asinoides* L.

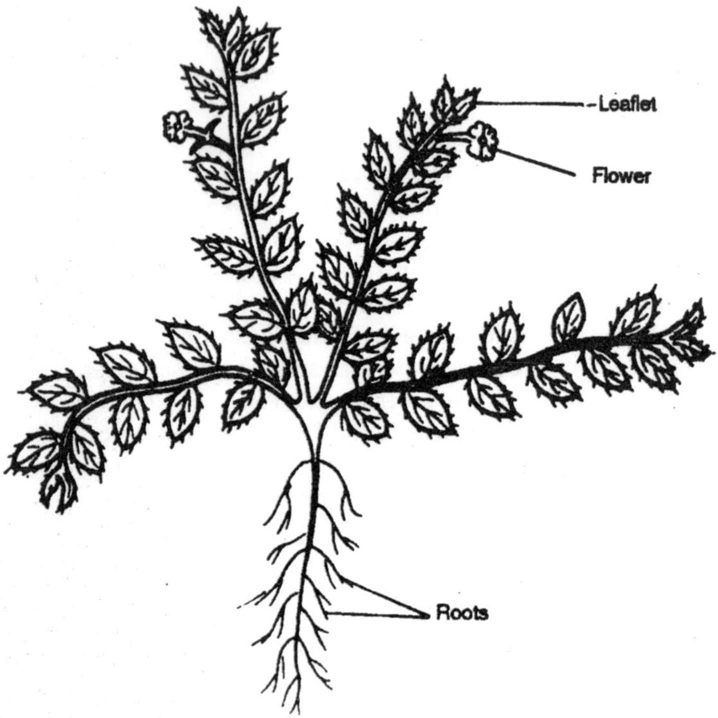

Shankhpushpi

Sesame seed

Sesame (Sesamum indicum) is a crop grown primarily for its oil-rich seeds. The small, cream-white sesame seed is used whole in cooking for its rich nutty flavour, and also yields a cooking oil. Sesame seeds are sometimes added to bagels and the top of hamburger buns. Sesame seeds are baked into crackers, often in the form of sticks. Sesame plants are also known as til in India and benne in Africa.

Sesame seeds can be made into a paste called tahini (used in hummus) and a Turkish confection called halvah. In sections of the Middle East and East Asia, popular treats are made from sesame mixed with honey or syrup and roasted (called pasteli in Greece). Sesame flavor (through oil and seeds (roasted and plain)) are also very popular in Korean cuisine. You can also see sesame seeds sprinkled onto some Sushi style foods.

East Asian cuisines, like Chinese cuisine uses sesame seeds and oil in some dishes, such as the dim sum dish, sesame seed balls.

Japanese cuisine uses sesami seeds to make *goma-dofu* which is made from sesami paste and ivy root powder.

The seeds are rich in Manganese, Copper and Calcium, and also contain Vitamin B1 - Thiamine.

Service Life

The life expectancy or number of cycles for which a processing unit will maintain its performance.

Sex Chromosomes

Those whose content is different in the two sexes - usually labeled X and Y (or W and Z), female sex has XX (or WW), male is XY (or WZ).

Shavegrass (Horsetail herb)

Stabilizes and strengthens lung membranes; effective in healing urinary tract infections.

Shepherd's purse (Capsella bursa-pastoris)

lowers blood pressure; reduces heavy menstrual flow (menorrhagia)70; reduces the incidence of hemorrhage in childbirth; heals urinary tract irritation and clears blood from the urine; stimulates uterine contractions71.

Shielded Metal-Arc Welding (SMAW)

An arc welding process that produces coalescence of metals by heating them with an arc between a covered metal electrode and the work. Shielding is obtained from decomposition of the electrode covering. Pressure is not used and filler metal is obtained from the electrode.

Shiitake Mushroom (Lentinus edodes)

Helps Immune system.

Shatavari

The drug consists of dried tuberous roots of *Asparagus racemosus* wild.

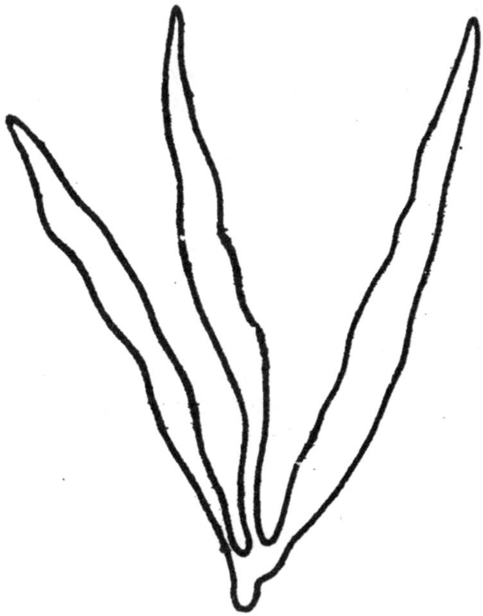

Shatavari

Shotgun Method

Sequencing method that involves randomly sequencing tiny cloned pieces of the genome, with no foreknowledge of where on a chromosome the piece originally came from. This can be contrasted with "directed" strategies, in which pieces of DNA from adjacent stretches of a chromosome are sequenced. Direct strategies eliminate the need for complex reassembly techniques. Because there are advantages to both strategies, researchers expect to use both random (or shotgun) and directed strategies in combination to sequence the human genome.

Signed (signature)

The record of who performed a particular action or review. This record may be initials, full handwritten signature, personal seal, or authenticated and secure electronic signature.

Significant

In a scientific study, significant means that a statistical analysis of the results has ruled out chance variation as the cause of an observed effect.

Sickle-cell Anemia

An inherited, potentially lethal disease in which a defect in hemoglobin, the oxygen-carrying pigment in the blood, causes distortion (sickling) and loss of red blood cells, producing damage to organs throughout the body.

Silica Silicon

Dioxide (SiO2) and its hydrated forms are classified as reactive and nonreactive. Generally, reactive Silica is removed by the anion exchange resin. Reactive Silica is only slightly ionized and is held lightly by the anion resin. It is for this reason that Silica is the first thing to break through when the resin nears exhaustion. Nonreactive Silica is generally considered to be particulate (colloidal) in nature.

Silk

Silk is a fibre made from the cocoons of *Bombyx mori* Linn.

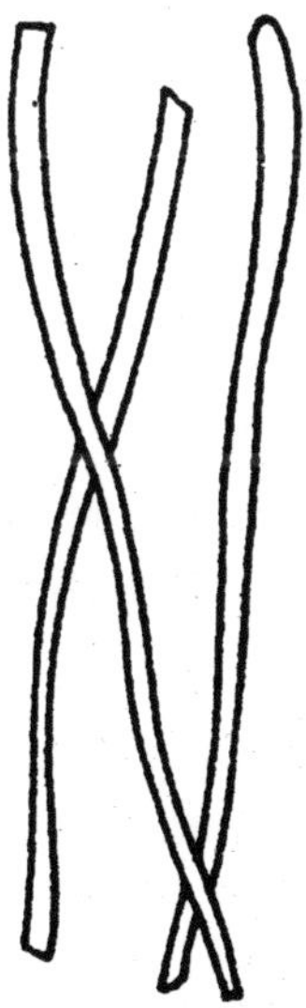

Silk fibre

Single Gene Disorder

Hereditary disorder caused by a mutant allele of a single gene (e.g., Duchenne muscular dystrophy, retinoblastoma, sickle cell disease).

Slippery elm (Ulmus fulva)

Demulcent; soothes damaged tissue; treats gastritis and ulcers; very effective for coughs72; very effective for sore throat73; diarrhea; sores74; remedy for broken bones; anti-inflammatory for the stomach.contraindicated during pregnancy.

Slope

An incline or deviation from the horizontal. A tube or pipe installed in the horizontal plane is said to slope if one end is positioned higher than the other.

Smoke Control

The use of physical barriers and mechanical ventilation to control the spread of smoke from a fire.

Smoke Purge

The use of mechanical ventilation to remove smoke resulting from fire.

Smoke Test

Visualization of airflow streams in a clean space using artificially generated smoke, such as Titanium smoke, CO2, or glycol fog.

Softener

Water treatment equipment that uses a sodium-based ion-exchange resin, principally to remove cations.

Softening

A pretreatment process which uses cation exchange resin to remove hardness elements (calcium and magnesium) from water. The cation resin is regenerated with Sodium Chloride (NaCl) and during the exchange process, the calcium and magnesium are removed from the water and replaced with sodium ions (Na+). The resulting sodium salts are much more soluble and do not precipitate, which provides better feed water to the RO system.

Software

An executable program that operates on an automated system.

Soldering

A metal joining process wherein coalescence is produced by heating to suitable temperatures and by using a nonferrous alloy fusible at temperatures below 427°C (800°F) and having a melting point below that of the base metals being joined. The filler metal is distributed between closely fitted surfaces of the joint by capillary attraction. In general, solders are lead-tin alloys and may contain antimony, bismuth, and other elements.

Solid extract

Solid or semisolid extracts prepared from native extracts by adjusting to the correct strength with suitable diluents.

Solid Tumors

Cancer cells which grow as a solid mass.

Soluble Antigen

Generally used in reference to vaccine production. As opposed to a whole live or attenuated virus, a soluble antigen is a fragment of the virus that produces immunity. Also refers to large molecular weight polysaccharides from some bacteria which can act as vaccines.

Solute

The substance that dissolves to form ions in solution.

Solvent

A liquid capable of dissolving a solute.

Solvent

An inorganic or organic liquid used as a vehicle for the

preparation of solutions or suspensions in the manufacture of an intermediate or API (Active Pharmaceutical Ingredient).

Somatic Cell

Any cell in the body except gametes and their precursors.

Somoclonal Variation

Genetic variation produced from the culture of plant cells from a pure breeding strain; the source of the variation is not known.

SOP (Standard Operating Procedures)

The description of necessary activities to respond to normal and abnormal situations in an operating system. The SOP may include a troubleshooting checklist, list of personnel to contact, etc. SOPs should also describe normal operation, maintenance, and cleaning of the system, and normal operating parameters. An SOP may be created for any system but an SOP must be created for each system requiring qualification.

Sorrel

The common sorrel, or spinach dock, is a perennial herb, which grows abundantly in meadows in most parts of Europe and is cultivated as a leaf vegetable. It is a slender plant about 60 cm high, with juicy stems and leaves. It has whorled spikes of reddish-green flowers, which bloom in June and July. The leaves are oblong, the lower ones being 7 to 15 cm in length, slightly arrow-shaped at the base, with very long petioles. The upper ones are sessile, and frequently become crimson.

As the flowers increase in size, they become a purplish colour. The stamens and pistils are on different plants. The seeds, when ripe, are brown and shining. The perennial roots run deeply into the ground.

The leaves of sorrel are eaten by the larvae of several species of Lepidoptera including blood-vein.

Common sorrel has been cultivated for centuries, although its popularity has decreased considerably over time. Because of the mildly acidic taste, it quenches thirst, and may be helpful in boosting the appetite. The leaves are edible and may be added to salads to sharpen the taste. They are often puréed in soups and sauces. The plant contains oxalic acid, which produces its characteristic flavour, and so may be contraindicated in people with rheumatic-type complaints, kidney or bladder stones, and the like. It is also a laxative.

Source Code

An original computer program either in human readable or machine-readable form.

Southern Blotting

Transfer by absorption of DNA fragments separated in electrophoretic gels to membrane filters for detection of specific base sequences by radiolabeled complementary probes.

Sparger

A device used to agitate, oxygenate, aerate, or add a chemical to a liquid by means of compressed air or gas entering through small holes in a pipe below the liquid surface.

Spearmint (Mentha spicata)

Antispasm; stomach.

Specific Conductance

The reciprocal of specific resistance usually expressed in micromhos/cm.

Specific Humidity

Also known as Humidity Ratio, and Absolute Humidity, is the weight of water vapor in each pound of dry air expressed in grains of moisture per pound of dry air, or pounds of moisture per pound of dry air. (also see: Saturation Humidity) NOTE: 7,000 grains = 1.0 pound. Humidity of air mixtures is normally discussed in terms of grains of moisture per pound rather than the more common term of relative humidity because the grains of moisture in an air stream do not change when it is heated or cooled, unless condensation takes place.

Specific Ion Determinations

Electrochemical measurement of trace ion levels in solution.

Specific Resistance

The resistance of a one-centimeter cube of water to the passage of electricity under standard conditions, expressed in ohms/cm. A measure of the Total Ionized Solids concentration.

Specific Volume

In Psychrometry, the cubic feet of the mixture per pound of dry air.

Specification

A list of testes, references to analytical procedures, and appropriate acceptance criteria that are numerical limits, ranges, or other criteria for the test described. It establishes the set of criteria to which an intermediate or API (Active Pharmaceutical Ingredient) should conform to be considered acceptable for its intended use. "Conformance to Specifications" means that the intermediate or API, when tested according to the listed analytical procedures, will meet the listed acceptance criteria.

Specificity

Exerting a definitive and distinctive influence on a particular part of the body and on the course of a particular disease.

Spikenard root (Aralia recemosa)

Diuretic; relieves coughs and asthma; Native Americans used it for menstrual irregularities; helps lung and kidney ailments.

Spinner Flasks

Small laboratory bioreactors used for the initial growth of mammalian cells lines.

Spore

A reproductive cell or seed of algae, fungi, or protozoa.

Spore, bacterial

A bacterial spore is a resistant body formed as part of the life cycle of some bacteria. Bacterial spores are able to withstand severe environmental conditions (e.g., heat, drying, chemicals) for many years. When conditions are favorable, spores germinate into vegetative bacterial cells capable of replication.

Sporicide

An agent that destroys bacterial and fungal spores.

Spray Drying

Process by which a material in suspension is converted into droplets that may be coated by a substance, either melted or dissolved in the droplet's media. The action in spray drying is primarily that of evaporation, energy is applied to the droplet forcing evaporation of the media with both energy and mass transfer through the droplet. Examples of this technology include, pharmaceutical tablet granulation, and rapid drying which results in free-flowing powders on a continuous basis. Spray drying process consists of the following steps:

1. Formation of a slurry to be sprayed; this slurry may be a simple concentrated solution or the dispersion of an insoluble material in a solution.
2. Liquid atomization into droplets; this action is critical as the droplet size will dictate the equipment size as well as the final product size. There are four types of atomization devices: air, airless, disk (or rotary) spray, and ultrasonic.
3. Exposure of the droplet to a heated gas flow; this gas (normally air) supplies the energy required to vaporize the solvent. Collection of the dry free-flowing powder or encapsulated liquid or solid.

Squaw vine (Mitchella repens)

Relieves painful menstruation; helps prevent miscarriage75; used during the last few weeks of pregnancy to aid childbirth.

Stable

A stable compound remains unchanged for a relatively long period of time.

Stability

Generally, stability refers to the physico-chemical condition of a parenteral, biological, or shelf life of labile drugs. Certain drugs must pass U.S.P. or CFR stability tests. For example, human serum albumin must pass certain limits of nephelometric turbidity. Also manufacturers must have documentation of potency of labile products under labeled storage conditions.

Stability Index

An empirical modification of the saturation index used to predict scaling or corrosive tendencies in water systems.

Star anise

Star anise is a spice that closely resembles anise in flavor, obtained from the star-shaped pericarp of Illicium verum, a native of N.E. China. It is widely used in Chinese cuisine, and to a lesser degree in South Asia and Indonesia. Star anise is an ingredient of the traditional five-spice powder of Chinese cooking. The seeds are sometimes chewed after meals to aid digestion.

Star anise contains anethole, the same ingredient which gives the unrelated anise its flavor. Recently, star anise has come into use in the West as a less expensive substitute for anise in baking as well as in liquor production.

Star anise has been used in a tea as a remedy for colic and rheumatism.

Japanese star anise (Illicium anisatum), a similar tree, is not edible because it is highly toxic; instead, it has been burned as incense in Japan. Cases of illness, including "serious neurological effects, such as seizures", reported after using star anise tea may be a result of using this species. Japanese star anise contains anisatin, which causes severe inflammation of the kidneys, urinary tract and digestive organs.

Stainless Steel

There are more than 70 standard types of stainless steel and many special alloys. These steels are produced in the wrought form (AISI types) and as cast alloys (ACI types). Generally, all are iron based, with 12 to 30 percent chromium, 0 to 22 percent nickel, and minor amounts of carbon, columbium, copper, molybdenum, selenium, tantalum, and titanium. There are three groups of wrought stainless steels:

1. Martensitic Alloys: characteristically magnetic and hardenable by heat treatment are oxidation resistant. They are exemplified by Type 410 (UNS S41000). Contain 12 to 20 percent chromium with controlled amount of carbon and other additives. Their corrosion resistance is inferior to austenitic stainless steels, and is generally used in mildly corrosive environments and for cutlery, turbine blades, and high-temperature parts.
2. Ferritic Stainless: characteristically magnetic but not hardenable by heat treatment. Contain 15 to as much as 30 percent Cr with low carbon content (0.1 percent). The higher chromium content improves its corrosive resistance. Type 430 (UNS S43000) widely used in nitric acid plants is a typical example. Corrosion resistance is rated good, although ferritic alloys are not good against reducing acids such as HCl.
3. Austenitic Stainless: widely used in bioprocessing, are characteristically non-magnetic, not hardenable by heat treatment, and are the most corrosion resistant of the three groups. These steels contain 16 to 26 percent chromium, 6 to 22 percent nickel. Carbon is kept low (0.08 percent) to minimize carbide precipitation. To avoid precipitation, special stainless steels stabilized with titanium, columbium, or tantalum, have been developed (types 321, 347, 348). Another approach to the problem is the use of low-carbon steels such as 304L and 316L, with 0.03 percent maximum carbon. Type 302 is the basic alloy of this group. Types 304 (UNS S30400) and 304L are low-carbon versions of 302. Types 316 (UNS S31600), 316L, and 317 (UNS S31700), with 2.5 to 3.5 percent molybdenum, are the most corrosion resistance.

Cast Stainless Alloys: are widely used in pumps, valves, and fittings. All corrosion resistant alloys have the letter C plus a second letter (A to N) denoting increasing nickel content. Numerals indicate maximum carbon. Typical members of this group are CF-8, similar to 304 stainless, CF-8M, similar to 316, and CD-4M Cu, which has improved resistance to nitric, sulfuric, and phosphoric acids.

Standard Atmospheric Conditions

At sea level these conditions are: 1. Temperature - 59°F. 2. Pressure - 29.921 Inches of mercury 3. Density - 0.0765 lbs dry air/cubic foot

Standard Dimensional Ratio (SDR)

The most commonly accepted means for providing a pipe wall thickness category and constant mechanical properties for many plastic materials. Used for solid, homogeneous pipe, the SDR is found by dividing the average outside diameter of a pipe by the wall thickness.

Standardize

To analyze a concentrated botanical extract so that predetermined levels of certain compounds (known as 'marker' compounds) are guaranteed to be present in every batch. These levels are generally chosen based on research results.

Standpipe System

A wet or dry system of piping, valves, outlets, and related equipment designed to provide water at specified pressures and installed exclusively for the fighting of fires.

Start-Up

The initial operation of equipment to prove that it is installed properly and operates as intended. Start-Up is considered complete when the selected equipment will adequately process product as specified.

State of Control

A condition in which all operating variables that affect performance remain within such ranges that the system or process performs consistently and as intended.

Steam distilling

In order to extract volatile or essential oils, plant material is either boiled in water or steam is passed through it. The volatiles are carried off in the steam and recovered in a condenser.

Steroidal Compounds

Steroids are a natural product class of widely distributed compounds. Steroids develop and control the reproductive tract in humans, molt insects, induce sexual reproduction in aquatic fungi. Therapeutically, steroids contribute cardiotonics (digitoxin), Vitamin D precursors, oral contraceptives (semi-synthetic progestins), antiinflammatory agents (corticosteroids) and anabolic agents (androgens).The phytochemical make up of this group of plant glycosides always includes a 4-membered hydrocarbon ring. This is true in animal-derived steroids and synthesized steroids as well.

In plants, steroidal content is divided into steroid saponins, which are very similar to triterpenoid saponins in the terpenoid group; or, they may be compounds which render them steroid alkaloids, from the alkaloid group(Harborne and Baxter, 290, 689). Steroidal compounds serve many functions both for the plant and also for humans: Combined steroids derived from plants have proven and continue to be valuable for medicinal purposes that range from topical antibiotics to relieving dysmenorrhea.

Stereoisomer

Two molecules are 'stereoisomers' of each other when they contain the exact same numbers and kinds of atoms, which are bonded to each other in the very same order; the only difference between them is the way certain bonds are oriented in space.

Statistical Process Control (SPC)

A process control method to demonstrate mathematically that a process or system is operating within the limitations established for the parameter(s) in question.

Steam In Place (also see: SIP)

Sterile Absence of life; usually refers to absence of viable microorganisms.

Sterile Water

For Injection, U.S.P. A form in which water is distributed in sterile packages. Sterile Water for Injection is intended mainly for use as a solvent for parenteral products such as sterile solids that must be distributed dry because of limited stability of their solutions. It must be packaged only in single-dose containers of not larger than 1-liter size.

Sterile Water for Irrigation, U.S.P.

This form of water meets most, but not all, of the requirements for Sterile Water for Injection. The exceptions are with respect of container size (i.e., the container may contain a volume of more than 1 liter), container design (i.e., the container may be designed so as to empty rapidly the contents as a single dose), particulate matter requirements (i.e., need not meet the requirement for Large Volume Injections for single-dose infusions), and labeling requirements (e.g., the designation "For Irrigation Only" and "Not For Injection" appear prominently on the label).

Sterile Engineering Design (Fermentation)

The application of techniques to prevent contamination of a fermentation process by undesirable organisms. It includes three basic phases relating to the operation of the plant. First, the fermenter with the ancillary equipment, pipework, and valves must be brought to a sterile state. Secondly, the fermenter feed must be sterilized, and finally, sterile barriers at the interface between the fermenter and the outside environment must be maintained.

Sterilization

The act or process, physical or chemical, that destroys or eliminates all viable microbes including resistant bacterial spores from a fluid or a solid. Despite being stated as an absolute, the action of sterilization is usually stated in terms of probability. Examples of sterilization methods are: steam treatment at 121°C, dry heat at 450°F, flushing with a sterilizing solution such as Hydrogen Peroxide (H2O2) or ozone (O3), irradiation, and filtration.

Sterilizing Filter

A filter that, when challenged with the microorganisms Brevundimonas diminuta, at a minimum concentration of 107 organisms per square centimeter of filter surface, produces a sterile effluent.

Steroid

An organic compound incorporating a perhydrocyclopentanophenanthrene nucleus.

2. Classified as lipids, naturally occurring steroids are hormones that are important regulators of animal development and metabolism at very low concentrations. A well known steroid, cholesterol, is present in membranes of animal tissues. Other steroids include testosterone (a male sex hormone), cortisone (an adrenocortical hormone), estrone (a female sex hormone), and progesterone.

Sterol

One of a group of fat-like substances found in animals, plants, fungi and microbes, which are alcohols with a cyclic nucleus known to chemists as perhydrocyclopentanophenanthrene.

Stevia Herb (Stevia rebaudiana)

Digestion, herb has very sweet taste.

Stomachic

Stimulates the action of the stomach.

Strain

A population of cells all descended from a single cell.

Strength

The concentration of the drug substance (for example, weight/weight, weight/volume, or unit dose/volume basis), and/or the potency, that is, the therapeutic activity of the drug product as indicated by appropriate laboratory tests or by adequately developed and controlled clinical data (expressed, for example, in terms of units by reference to a standard).

Structure-activity relationship

The influence of structural features, such as the conformation of the drug molecule and optical and geometric isomerism, on the pharmacologic activity of the drug molecule.

Study design

A placebo is an inactive substance given to one group of subjects, with the active substance being given to another group of subjects; then the results between the test and placebo group are compared. In a double-blind clinical trial of a drug, the researchers administering the test substances do not know which subjects receive the placebo, and which receive the active substance, until the conclusion of the study. Then the study is said to be "randomised, placebo-controlled, double-blind," meaning the subjects receiving the placebo or test substance were randomly chosen; the comparison is made between the test substance and a placebo, an inactive substance; and neither the subjects, not the investigators, know which subjects were given placebo until the study is concluded. This type of study is usually considered to have the most scientific credibility, because it prevents the expectations of the investigators, or subjects, from affecting the outcome. A variation on this is the double-blind, placebo-controlled, cross-over study, in which only one study groups is compared; some subjects receive placebo, and others the active substance; then, the treatment is reversed, and in the next phase of the study, the subjects that received placebo are given the active substance, and those that were given active substance receive the placebo.

Sublimation

The process of vaporizing a solid substance by heat and then condensing it (without its having passed through a liquid state in either direction), a process of purification by separating the nonvaporizable impurities, a process analogous to the distillation of liquids.

Submerged Arc Welding (SAW)

An arc welding process that produces coalescence of metals by heating them with an arc or arcs between a bare metal electrode or electrodes and the work. A blanket of granular, fusible material on the work shields the arc. Pressure is not used and filler metal is obtained from the electrode and sometimes from a supplemental source (welding rod, flux, or metal granules).

Substrate

Reactive material - the substance on which an enzyme acts.

Subsurface Carbon Enrichment

In metals, a rise in the carbon signal at depths from 15 to 20 angstroms (Å). This indicates that organic material is buried in cracks, crevices, pits, or smeared material. Subsurface carbon is most commonly found in materials having rough morphology generally associated with machining processes.

Sulfide

An organic compound containing sulfur bonded to carbon; monosulfide: R-C-S-C-R; disulfide: R-C-S-S-C-R; Trisulfide: R-C-S-S-S-C-R (mono=one, di=two, tri=3; R= R group.)

Sulfoxide

An organic compound containing a sulfur atom bonded to an oxygen atom.

Sumac

Rhus is a genus of woody shrubs and trees, all with the leaves spirally arranged and pinnately compound (some species are trifoliate). The flowers are in dense panicles or spikes 5-30 cm long, each flower very small, creamy white, greenish or red, with five petals. The fruit form dense clusters of reddish drupes. Commonly called sumac or sumach, the approximately 250 species of Rhus are placed in the family Anacardiaceae. Some species (including poison ivy, poison oak, and poison sumac), often placed in this genus, are here treated in the genus Toxicodendron, which have grayish-white fruit. The name derives from the Greek name for sumac, rhous.

Supernatant

The material floating on the surface of a liquid mixture (often the liquid component that has the lowest density).

Surface Finishes

This term shall apply to all interior surface finishes accessible and inaccessible, that directly or indirectly come in contact with the designated product in bioprocessing equipment and distribution system components (ASME BPEa-2000). Final criteria shall be determined by Ra values rather than polishing methods.

For Piping, Tubing, and Fittings:

1. As fabricated
2. Pickled and/or passivated
3. Bright hydrogen annealed
4. Mechanically polished
5. Mechanically buffed
6. Chemically polished
7. Electropolished

For Sheet, Strip, and Plate:

1. As fabricated. Without any specific surface treatments.
2. Rolled Finish. Manufactured by either hot or cold rolled process.
3. No. 1. A dull, hot rolled finish, annealed and pickled.
4. No. 2D. A dull, cold rolled finish, annealed and pickled.
5. No. 2B. A bright, cold rolled finish, annealed and pickled.
6. No. 4. A general purpose polished finish widely used for architectural panels, trim, and sanitary equipment. Following initial grinding with coarse abrasives, the surface is finally finished with lubricated 150 grit abrasive belts.
7. No. 4S. Processed as No. 4 except the final surface is polished to a smother finish. The purchaser must specify this alternative finish; the specification must state a No. 4 finish, using a 240 or 320 grit mechanical polish, whose particular surface roughness must meet the specified Ra value.
8. No. 6. A dull finish having a lower reflectivity than No. 4. It is produced by a tampico brushing in a medium of abrasive and oil and is used primarily for architectural applications.
9. No. 7. A finish with a high degree of reflectivity, produced by buffing to a finely ground surface without removing the grit lines.
10. No. 8. The most reflective finish, obtained by polishing with successively finer abrasives and buffing extensively with very fine buffing rouges. This finish is most widely used for press plates, mirrors, etc.

For Wrought and Cast Forgings:

1. As fabricated or machined
2. Mechanically ground, polished, or buffed
3. Abrasive blast cleaned, using one of the following methods:
   a. Sand blast

   b. Shot blast
   c. Glass blast
   d. Wet blast
4. Slurry polished
5. Roll deburred
6. Chemically cleaned
   a. Acid washed (pickled and passivated)
   b. Solvent washed
7. Electropolished

Surface Iron Oxide Layer

Surface iron oxide layer present when the 316L stainless steel's iron composition signal is higher than its chromium signal at the surface.

Surface Residual

A foreign substance that adheres to a surface by chemical reaction, adhesion, adsorption, or ionic bonding (for example, corrosion, rouging, and staining).

Surface Texture

The repetitive or random deviations of the nominal metal surface from the three-dimensional topography of the surface. Surface texture includes roughness, waviness, lay, and flaws.

Surface Water

Any water where the source is above ground such as rivers, lakes, and reservoirs. Surface waters are usually higher in suspended matter and organic material and lower in dissolved minerals than well water.

Surfactant

Any substance that changes the nature of a surface, such as lowering the surface tension of water.

Suspended Solids

Undissolved solids that can be removed by filtration. Determined by a filter paper before and after filtration of a water sample.

Suspension

A specific category of pharmaceutical product that must be in a colloidal dispersion (suspension) for proper action. For example, Kaolin/Pectin works as an adsorbant because its high surface area in suspension.

Sustainable

(Agriculture, logging, manufacturing, etc.) environmentally friendly methods that allow the continued production of a commodity without damage to the ecosystem. Includes soil, water supplies, biodiversity or other surrounding resources. Synergism- an interaction in which the effects of two in combination is greater than the sum of the singular effects.

Synthetic

Compounds produced by total synthesis from unrelated and base reactants.

Semi-Synthetic

Compounds produced by a chemical modification of a natural product.

Superoxide, superoxide radical

A highly reactive form of oxygen, the superoxide anion, produced when oxygen is reduced by a single electron. Produced as a by product of certain metabolic reactions.

Symbiosis

The phenomenon of two entities performing a joint function that neither entity can perform alone.

Synergistic

Acting together. In botanical medicine, the notion that therapeutic efficacy results from the combined actions of multiple active constituents, rather than a single constituent.

Synergy

In medicinal plants, constituents that somehow work together are said to be working in 'synergy' or 'synergistically.' Two or more constituents may result in an increased effect (potentiating synergy), or one constituent may modify the toxic effects of another (attenuating synergy); protective synergy is when one constituent stabilizes or protects another (i.e., an antioxidant may prevent the breakdown of another constituent). Synergy is thought to occur in addition to any additive effects the constituents of an herb may have (simplified as 1 + 1 > 2). Another type of synergy occurs when one constituent produces an effect upon an organism that allows a separate constituent to have an enhanced effect on that organism. For example, some herbs that produce the antimicrobial alkaloid berberine also produce a chemical that inhibits bacteria from pumping the berberine out of their cells. Some herbs (i.e., Valerian) do not have a prominent 'active ingredient' but instead achieve their effects through synergy of multiple constituents. Synergy can be found operating in formulas as well; for example, Nettle root & Pygeum bark work better together for BPH (benign prostatic hyperplasia) than either herb alone. Although the word synergy can have several definitions, there is a specific mathematical test for true synergistic interactions between constituents, known as the 'isobole method.'

Synthesis

Creating products through chemical and enzymatic reactions.

System Specifications

Descriptions of how the system will meet the functional requirements.

Szechuan pepper

The Szechuan peppercorn (Zanthoxylum piperitum, Zanthoxylum simulans, Zanthoxylum sancho and some other species in the genus Zanthoxylum) is not a member of the pepper family. It is the outer pod of the tiny fruit of a plant related to the pricklyash.

It is known in Chinese as □□ *h uājiāo (faa1jiu1* in some dialects), literally "flower pepper"; a lesser-used name is □□ *shānjiāo,* "mountain pepper". In Japanese these same characters (□□) are pronounced *sanshō*, which can also be written in kana as □□□□□. In Tibetan, it is known as emma. It is widely used in the cuisine of Sìchuân province, from which it takes its name (Sìchuân used to be spelt Szechuan).

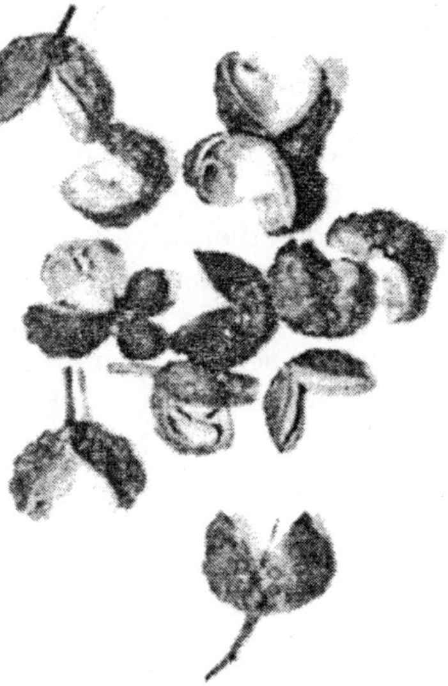

The taste of Szechuan peppercorns is not hot like black or red pepper, but is a kind of tingly numbness (caused by its 3% of hydroxy-alpha-sanshool) that sets the stage for these hot spices. Recipes often suggest lightly toasting and then crushing the tiny seedpods before adding them to food. It is generally added at the last moment. Star aniseed and ginger are often used with it and it figures prominently in spicy Szechuan cuisine. It is considered to go well with fish, duck and chicken dishes. It is also available as an oil (marketed as either "Szechuan Pepper Oil" or "Hwajiaw Oil"). In this form it is best used in stir fry noodle dishes without hot spices. The preferred recipe includes ginger oil and brown sugar to be cooked with a base of noodles and vegetables, with rice vinegar and szechuan pepper oil to be added after cooking.

□□□ *(huājiāoyān)* is a mixture of salt and Szechuan pepper, roasted and browned in a wok and served as a condiment to accompany chicken, duck and pork dishes. The peppercorns can also be lightly fried in order to make a spicy oil with various uses.

Szechuan pepper is one of the few spices important for Tibetan and Bhutani cookery of the Himalayas, because few spices can be grown there. The national dish of Tibet are momos, a pasta stuffed with yak and flavoured with Szechuan pepper, garlic, ginger and onion. The noodles are steamed and served dry, together with a fiery sauce. Tibetans believe it can sanitize meat that may not be so fresh.

In Japan the dried and powdered leaves of Zanthoxylum sancho are used to make noodle dishes and soups mildly hot and fragrant. The whole leaves, □□□ kinome, are used to flavour vegetables, especially bamboo shoots, and to decorate soups.

Szechuan peppercorns are one of the traditional ingredients in the Chinese spice mixture five-spice powder and also shichimi togarashi, a Japanese seven-flavour seasoning.

T

Tamarind

The Tamarind is a tropical tree, originally from east Africa but now introduced into most of tropical Asia as well as Latin America. The tree can grow up to 20 meters in height, and stays evergreen in regions without a dry season. Tamarind timber consists of hard, dark red heartwood and softer, yellowish sapwood. The leaves consist of 10 to 18 leaflets. The tree produces brown pod-like fruits, which contain pulp and hard-coated seeds. The seeds can be scarified to enhance germination.

The pulp of the fruit is used as a spice both in Asian as well as in Latin American cuisine, and is also an important ingredient to Worcestershire sauce and HP sauce. The pulp of a young fruit is very sour, and hence suitable for main dishes, whereas a ripened fruit is sweeter and can be used in desserts, drinks, or as a snack. The pulp, leaves, and the bark also have medical applications. For example, in the Philippines, the leaves have been traditionally used in herbal tea for reducing malaria fever. Due to its denseness and durability, tamarind heartwood can be used in making furniture and wood flooring. Tamarind trees are very common in South India particularly in Andhra Pradesh. They are used to provide shade on the country roads and highways like oak trees. Monkeys love the ripened tamarind fruit. It is a staple in the South Indian diet, where it is used to prepare Sambhar (spicy lentil soup with lots of vegetables), Pulihora rice, and various types of chutneys.

Tamarind is available in Indian stores worldwide. It is also sold as a candy in Mexico.

T cell

Lymphoid cells from the bone marrow, which migrate to the thymus gland and develop into mature lymphocytes; syn: T lymphocytes.

Tangential Flow Filtration

A separation method that transfers components of one system (stream) into another. The stream the product is being extracted from crosses the stream that the product is being transferred to, multiple times.

Tannin

Acidic substances found in the bark of certain plants. Tannins are divided into two classes, condensed tannins and hydrolysable tannins.

Taxonomy

The development of approaches to organize and summarize our knowledge about the variety or organisms that exist.

Tay-Sachs Disease

An inherited disease of infancy characterized by profound mental retardation and early death; it is caused by a recessive gene mutation.

T-Cell (T-lymphocyte)

A blood cell, probably originating from bone marrow, but which matures in the thymus. Some T-cells are responsible for cell-mediated immunity and in the production of antibodies. Telomere The end of a chromosome. This specialized structure is involved in the replication and stability of linear DNA molecules.

Team Biologics

A partnership between FDA's Office of Regulatory Affairs (ORA) and CBER to focus on inspectional and compliance issues in biologics. Its goal is to ensure the quality and safety of biologic products and resolve inconsistencies.

Temperature

A specific degree of heat intensity. There are three temperature designations associated with psychrometrics: 1. Dry Bulb (DB) - The air temperature as measured by a standard thermometer. 2. Wet Bulb (WB) - The air temperature measured by a thermometer with its reservoir bulb wrapped in a moistened cloth wick and exposed to an air stream moving at a velocity of 1,000 feet per minute. 3. Dewpoint temperature (DP) - Also called Saturation Temperature is the temperature at which condensation of moisture begins (air is holding 100% of the moisture it can) when the air is cooled, measured in °F.

Teratogenic compounds

Compounds which have profound effects on developmental stages of an organism.

Terminal Sterilization

The process applied to product sealed in its final container that transforms a non-sterile product into a sterile one.

Terminal Sterilization

This term is a gross misnomer because it refers specifically to the terminal heat sterilization of LVPs usually by steam.

Terminally Ill

For an individual, it means that the subject has a life expectancy of six months or less as stated in writing by his or her attending physician and surgeon.

Terpenoids

Terpenoids form the largest group of plant products and are the most common ingredient in volatile oils. They include camphor, Beta-carotene, and digitalin, for example, and are sometimes referred to as isoprenoids, due to the fact that all terpenoids are derived from a 5-carbon precursor isoprene. Terpenoids are categorized as monoterpenoids and monoterpenoid lactones, sesquiterpenoids and sesquiterpenoid lactones, diterpenoids, and triterpenoids. Of these four groups, triterpenoids forms the largest. Carotenoids are formed through a head-to-tail combination of geranylgeranyl pyrophosphate, the same precursor to monoterpenoids.

Monoterpene, sesquiterpene, and diterpene alkaloids, as well as steroidal alkaloids, are classified as alkaloids due to the presence of nitrogen in their structure. Despite that classification, those alkaloids, and some phenols as well (for instance, rotenone), may contain terpenoidal atoms or compounds or isoprenoid derivatives.

Monoterpenoids have a head-to-tail formation of their ten-carbon precursor, geranyl pyrophosphate. These constituents are present in volatile oils. Monoterpenoids often have a strong smell; they are the source of such scents as spearmint (carvone), bergamot and lavendar (both of which contain linalyl acetate), and sweet rose (nerol). Monoterpenoids occur in insect pheromones as well. Monoterpenoids vary in pharmacological use, as expectorants, anthelmintics, anticholesteremics, insecticides, and antiseptics.

The phrase bitter principles, which refers to the bitter-tasting monoterpenoid lactones known as iridoids are also components of volatile oils and have been used to stimulate actions within the body, such as mucosal or gastric secretion. The attachment of a glucose to a hydroxyl group on the lactone ring is the determining factor in recognizing a lactone. These isoflavonoid polyphenols are sometimes also referred to as iridoid glycosides, because they are often present in glycosidic form. Iridoids usually occur in angiosperms, especially valerian, gentian, blue flag, and orris root, and can have, aside from the therapeutic actions described above, antimicrobial and antileukemic properties.

Sesquiterpenoids occur with monoterpenoids in plant essential oils, especially in the families Labiatae, Myrtaceae, Pinaceae, and Rutaceae. They also occur in micro-organisms, marine animals, fighting insects, and insect pheromonal secretions. Some are very toxic, but sesquiterpenes can be used as antifungals, carminatives, insecticides, or as an antibiotic. This latter action has been successfully demonstrated against staphylococcus areus and candida albicans, by sesquiterpenes found in marine alga. A sesquiterpenes found in chamomile, is an antiinflammatory agent.

With the addition of a y-lactone sesquiterpenoids become sesquiterpene lactones such as those found in absynthe and arnica. The cytotoxicity of sesquiterpene lactones prevents their widespread use but encourages research into antitumor applications. Often these are the components causing contact dermatitis and some are lethal (ibid.).

Many resin acids, termed diterpenoid acids are included in this group, as are plant hormones called gibberellins. Many of the diterpenoids are toxic, similar to sesquiterpenoids, but some have antibiotic, antiviral, antiinflammatory, and bitter tonic uses (ibid). Ginkgolides, diterpenoids from the Ginkgo biloba plant, are fast becoming one of today's most highly-esteemed phytochemicals, finding use in the treatment of memory loss, allergies, asthma, brain injury, and more.

Triterpenoid saponins, or sapogenins, are plant glycosides which lather in water and are used in detergents, or as foaming agents or emulsifiers, and have enormous medical implications due to their antifungal, antimicrobial, and adaptogenic properties. Glycyrrhizin, from licorice root, is an example of a saponin used for antiinflammatory purposes in place of cortisone.

Steroid saponins are similar to the sapogenins and related to the cardiac glycosides. Therapeutically, steroidal saponins their ability to interact medically and beneficially with the cardiac glycosides, sex hormones, Vitamin D, and other factors, render these phytochemicals components of great medical significance. For instance, diosgenin, from Wild Yam, was used in the development of the first oral contraceptive.

Phytosterols are necessary to plant membranes and plant cell growth. Sitosterol, stigmasterol, and campesterol are the most common. It has been demonstrated that B-sitosterol decreases the risk of atherosclerosis by lowering plasma concentrations of LDL's (low-density lipoproteins). Ergosterol, combined with ultra violet light, becomes vitamin D2. Vitamin D3, mentioned in the first issue of The Protocol Journal of Botanical Medicines as a topical treatment for psoriasis, is obtained from 7-dehydrocholesterol.

Carotenoids, or forty-carbon tetraterpenoids, are lipid-soluble terpenes found in all forms of plants. Their value to animals comes from the splitting of the C40 molecule into the twenty-carbon isoprenoid alcohol known as Vitamin A, a process which occursafter the substance has been ingested.

Test Procedure

A sequence of activities which when executed successfully provides documentary evidence that part of the system works as specified.

Theoretical Yield

The quantity that would be produced at any appropriate phase of manufacture, processing, or packing of a particular drug product, based upon the quantity of components to be used, in the absence of any loss or error in actual production.

Thermophile

An organism that grows best at greater than 50°C (122°F).

Thermophilic (Of A Microorganism)

With optimum temperature for growth above 45°C, many thermophilic bacteria exist at high temperatures (greater than 80°C) and many of their enzymes which posses high thermal stability, are of great commercial interest.

Thiosulfinate

An organic compound containing two sulfur atoms bonded together, one of which is also double-bonded to an oxygen atom. Example: allicin.

Thrombin (Blood Coagulation Factor II)

An enzyme (the activated thrombogen) formed in the blood, after this is shed, that converts fibrinogen into fibrin for clot formation. It is formed from conjunction of prothrombin and calcium salts. It is also a sterile protein substance prepared from prothrombin of bovine origin through interaction with thromboplastin in the presence of calcium. Bovine thrombin is often used to aid production of serum from "salvage" plasma.

Thrombosis

Clotting within a blood vessel that may cause infarction of tissues supplied by the vessel.

Throughput Volume

The amount of solution passed through an exchange bed before the resin is exhausted.

A pyrimidine component of nucleic acid first isolated from the thymus.

Thyme (Thymus vulgaris)

Reduces bacteria growth; reduces mucous in the lungs; eliminates hookworms in the intestines; strengthens the nervous system.

Time Stamp

A part of the audit trail that clearly documents the sequence of events in human terms, helping to authenticate an electronic signature and minimizing the chances of signer repudiation. A local time stamp correlates with the whereabouts of the signer. With client-server data systems used by international companies and records accessed from remote sites (such as on business trips), time stamps that reflect the local time of only the user might make the sequence of actions for an individual record appear inconsistent. For example, the approval by a peer reviewer could be signed at 9:00 a.m. on a chromatographic analysis that was performed at 11:00 a.m. in a different time zone. Local time stamps should probably be supplemented consistently with the time stamp of a remote server, with one stamp clearly labeled as local.

Tincture of Iodine

A germicidal solution of iodine in aqueous alcohol used primarily as antiseptic on skin and tissue.

Tissue Culture

Growing mammalian cells in the laboratory in a tissue culture medium (in vitro). For example, this allows researchers to determine the effects of various chemicals on mammalian cells without experimenting directly on live animals or man. Since a molecule of some toxic substances can harm a single mammalian cell, even one part-per-billion of some impurities can affect a tissue culture. Therefore, water used to make up tissue culture media should be extremely pure.

Titer

A measured sample - the strength of a solution or the concentration of a substance (as an antibody) in solution as determined by titration.

Titration

Volumetric analysis by means of the addition of definite amounts of a test solution to a solution of a known amount of the substance analyzed.

TNT (Tumor Necrosis Therapy)

Therapeutic agents that target dead and dying cells found primarily at the core of the tumor.

Toe of Weld

The junction between the face of a weld and the base material.

Tolerance

Capacity for enduring a large amount of a substance (food, drug, or poison) without an adverse effect, and showing decreased sensitivity to subsequent doses of the substance. With medications, tolerance can lead to gradual loss of effectiveness.

2. Failure to mount an immune reaction on exposure to what would normally be an antigenic substance.

Ton of Refrigeration

A unit used to indicate the size of a refrigeration unit. One ton of refrigeration effect is equivalent to removing 12,000 Btu/hr of heat, or melting one ton of ice in a 24-hour period.

Tobacco

Tobacco consists of leaves and herb of *Nicotiana tabacum* Linn.

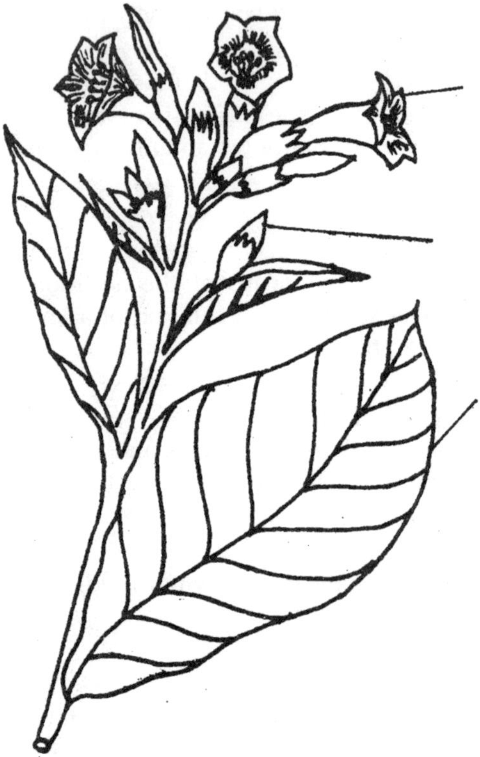

Tobacco

Tonic

A medicine that increases strength and tone.

Topical

A medication applied to the skin, an ointment. Usually a medicament suspended in a carrier such as petrolatum or another oil based carrier. Filtration at elevated temperatures is usually possible.

Topical Product

A pharmaceutical product meant to be applied to the skin or soft tissue in the form of liquid, cream, or ointment, and therefore needs not be aseptic. Sterile ophthalmic products throughout are manufactured aseptically.

Total Bacteria Count

An estimation of the total number of bacteria in a sample based usually on Standard Methods procedures for collecting, incubating, and counting colony-forming units (cfu).

Total Dissolved Solids (TDS) The term used to describe inorganic ions in the water. Usually measured by electrical conductance of the water corrected to 25°C, and expressed as ppm (parts per million).

Total Heat (TH)

The sum of sensible heat and latent heat.

Total Ionized Solids

Concentration of dissolved ions in solution expressed in concentration units of Sodium Chloride (NaCl). It determines the operating life of ion exchange resins and is calculated from measurements of Specific Resistance.

Total Organic Carbon (TOC)

A measure of the level of organic impurities in water by their carbon content that determines the operating life of activated carbon beds. This is one of the parameters used to determine the purity of Semiconductor Grade water. Feed water will have TOC measured in ppm (parts per million), and ultrapure water (UPW) will have TOC measured in ppb (parts per billion).

Total Solids

Total solids in water include both dissolved and suspended solids. Determined by weighing sample before and after evaporation.

Toxic

Pertaining to a substance that is harmful.

Toxic chemical

Substances that can cause severe illness, poisoning, birth defects, disease or death when ingested, inhaled or absorbed by organisms.

Toxic molecules

Molecules which result in abnormal physiological, metabolic or developmental function.

Toxicology

The scientific study of toxic substances, including their chemistry, pharmacology, and prevention and treatment of exposure to toxins.

2. A science that deals with poisons, their effects, and the problems involved.

Toxicity Characteristic Leaching Procedure (TCLP)

Test to determine when a waste is hazardous or requires treatment to become less hazardous; useful in monitoring treatment techniques.

Toxin

A substance produced by microorganisms that can inhibit cell growth in tissue culture and may cause temperature rise in animals.

2. Any poisonous agent, especially a poisonous substance produced by one living organism that is poisonous to other organisms. Toxins are usually very unstable, notably toxic when introduced into the tissues, and typically capable of inducing antibody formation.

Toxoid

An antigenic toxin. Example is tetanus toxoid that is a bacterial vaccine.

TPA (Tissue Plasminogen Activator)

A recombinant drug used in the management of heart attacks to prevent clotting. Produced by Genentech and one of the first successful recombinant DNA drugs to be commercialized.

Trace Analysis

Analyzing constituents present in ppm and ppb concentrations. Trace analysis requires extremely pure reagents, made with ultrapure Type I reagent grade water.

Traceability

A prerequisite for trustworthy records, apart from data security. Traceability is the part of the laboratory data system audit trail that holds the evidence of who did what to a record and when.

Tracer

A radioactively labeled nucleic acid component included in a reassociation reaction in amounts too small to influence the progress of reaction.

Traditional Chinese Medicine (TCM)

A system of ethnomedicine based on the use of herbal medicines and other therapies originating and derived from Chinese folk medicine. Key concepts in TCM are harmony with nature, the five elements, and balance between yin and tang.

Transcription

The process by which the genetic information encoded in the gene, represented as a linear sequence of deoxyribonucleotides (DNA), is copied into an exactly complementary sequence of ribonucleotides known as mRNA (messenger RNA).

Transduction

The transfer of genetic material from one cell to another by means of a viral vector (for bacteria, the vector is Bacteriophage).

Transfection

The acquisition of new genetic markers by addition of viral DNA to cells.

Transfer Panel

A panel to which process and utilities are piped, allowing

cross connections between different use points. A jumper spool is used to connect the desired process/utility users and mechanically preclude erroneous connections to other lines.

Transfer RNA (tRNA)

A class of RNA having structures with triplet nucleotide sequences that are complementary to the triplet nucleotide coding sequences of mRNA. The role of tRNAs in protein synthesis is to bond with amino acids and transfer them to the ribosomes, where proteins are assembled according to the genetic code carried by mRNA.

Transfer Systems

Equipment allowing the introduction and removal of material, toxic and/or sterile, with continuous protection to both operator and product.

Transformation

A process by which the genetic material carried by an individual cell is altered by incorporation of exogenous DNA into its genome.

Transformation products

Chemicals that are derived from a particular compound when it undergoes chemical changes during extraction, processing, or spontaneous decomposition.

Transgenics

The alteration of a plant or animal's DNA such that it contains a gene from another organism. There are two types of cells in animal and plants, germ line cells (the sperm and egg in animals, pollen and ovule in plants) and somatic cells (all other cells). Transgenic animals have alterations in their germ line DNA so the alterations are passed on to the offspring. That is done to produce therapeutics, to study disease, and to improve farm animals. Transgenic plants have been created for increased resistance to disease and insects as well as to make biopharmaceuticals.

Translation

The process in which the genetic code carried by mRNA directs the synthesis of proteins from amino acids.

Treatment Investigational New Drug

An Investigational New Drug that makes a promising new drug available to desperately ill patients as early in the drug development process as available. FDA permits the drug to be used if there is preliminary evidence of efficacy and it treats a serious or life-threatening disease, or if there is not comparable therapy available.

Triglyceride

Combinations of glycerol with three of five different fatty acids; syn: triacylglycerols or neutral fats.

Trihalomethanes

Compounds present in the feed water that are formed by the reaction of Chlorine and the organic material in the water. Activated carbon and degasification can reduce THMs.

Triterpenes

A class of terpenoid substances based on a 30 carbon structure, Triterpenoids are widespread in plants and include many saponins and sterols.

Tube Size

Tube is sized by its nominal outside diameter. For bioprocessing equipment, tube does not include pipe.

Tumor

An abnormal growth of cells. Also defined as a circumscribed growth, not inflammatory in character, arising from preexisting tissue, but independent of the normal rate or laws of growth of such tissue, and subserving no physiological function.

Tumor Pathogenesis

Morphological and physiological changes associated with tumor growth.

Tumor-Suppressor Genes

Genes that normally restrain cell growth but, when missing or inactivated by mutation, allow cells to grow uncontrolled.

Tulsi

The plant of Tulsi is an annual herb with much branched stem having verticillate inflorescence. The flowers are purple in colour in recemes.

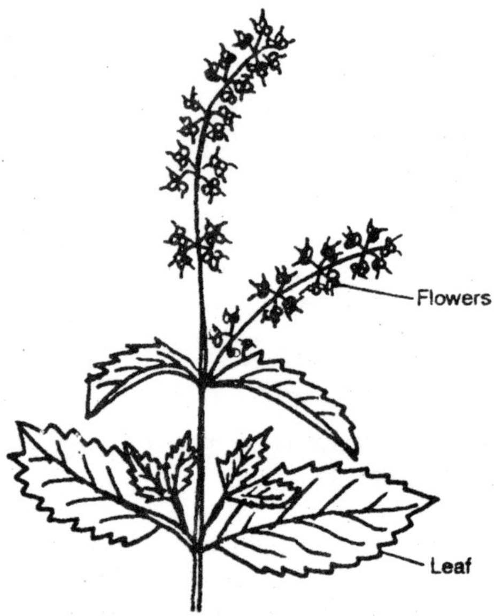

Tulsi plant

Turbidity

A suspension of fine particles that obscures light rays but requires many days for sedimentation because of small particle size.

Turmeric

Turmeric (*Curcuma longa,* also known as tumeric or curcumin) is a spice commonly used in curries and other south Asian cooking. It is a significant ingredient in most commercial curry powders. Turmeric is also used to give a yellow color to some prepared mustards, canned chicken broth, and other foods, and is also used as a fabric dye.

Turmeric is a member of the ginger family, Zingiberaceae.

In traditional medicine, turmeric is thought to have many healthful properties. It is taken in some Asian countries as a dietary supplement, which allegedly helps with stomach problems and other ailments. It is popular served as a tea in Okinawa, Japan.

A 2004 UCLA-Veterans Affairs study involving genetically altered mice suggests that curcumin, the yellow pigment in curry spice, might inhibit the accumulation of destructive beta amyloids in the brains of Alzheimer's patients and also break up existing plaques. "Curcumin has been used for thousands of years as a safe anti-inflammatory in a variety of ailments as part of Indian traditional medicine," Gregory Cole, Professor of medicine and neurology at the David Geffen School of Medicine at UCLA said.

It is also used in product systems that are packaged to protect them from sunlight. The oleoresin is used for oil-containing products. The curcumin/polysorbate solution or curcumin powder dissolved in alcohol is used for water containing products. Over-colouring, such as in pickles, relishes and mustard, is sometimes used to compensate for fading.

Turmeric has found application in canned beverages, baked products, dairy products, ice cream, yoghurts, yellow cakes, biscuits, popcorn-colour, sweets, cake icings, cereals, sauces, gelatines, direct compression tablets, etc. In combination with Annatto (E160b) it has been used to colour cheeses, dry mixes, salad dressings, winter butter and margarine.

Investigations into the low incidence of colorectal cancer amongst ethnic groups with a large intake of curries compared with the indigenous population have discovered that some active ingredients of turmeric may have anti-cancer properties. Second-stage trials of a turmeric-based drug as a possible treatment for cancer are currently underway.

Consuming large doses is not recommended in cases of gallstones, obstructive jaundice, acute bilious colic and toxic liver disorders.

Vicco Labs of India manufactures a popular skin cream formulated with turmeric cream, which it claims to "prevent the penetration of ultra violet rays of the sun into the skin." The Government of Thailand is funding a project to extract and isolate tetrahydrocurcuminoids (THC) from turmeric. THC are colorless compounds that might have antioxidant and skin lightening properties and might be used to treat skin inflammations, making these compounds useful in cosmetics formulations..

Active substance of turmeric is polyphenol curcumin, also known as C.I. 75300, or Natural Yellow 3. Systematic chemical name is (1E,6E)-1,7-bis(4-hydroxy-3-methoxyphenyl)-1,6-heptadiene-3,5-dione. It can exist at least in two tautomeric forms, keto and enol. The keto form is preferred in solid phase and the enol form in solution.

2. Turmeric consists of the prepared rhizomes of *Curcuma domestica.* Valeton.

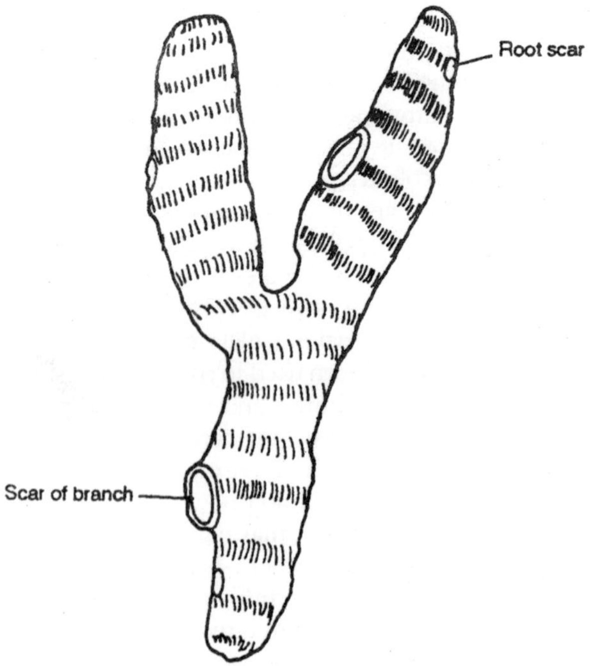

Turmeric

Turnover

Also known as "hand over" in the U.K. It is a formal transfer of custody for a system or unit to another group, department, or operating company.

Turnover Package (TOP)

A collection of pertinent design, construction, vendor, and operational documentation. This collection of documentation is used for the qualification and process validation activity, as well as reference and single source information for the life of any particular system, process, or piece of equipment.

Two-Bed Deionizer

Separate beds or layers of cation and anion exchange resins. Results in lower purity than mixed-bed deionization, but provides higher capacity in terms of throughput.

Tyrosine (Tyr)

A Phenolic alpha amino acid; a precursor of the hormones epinephrine, norepinephrine, thyroxine, and triiodothyronine, and of the black pigment melanin.

U

Ultra Low Penetration Air filters (ULPA)

Extended media dry filters in a rigid frame that have a minimum particle-collection efficiency of 99.999% for particles greater than or equal to 0.12μm in size. Most commonly used in microelectronics, few uses in pharmaceuticals.

Ultracentrifugation

The separation of macromolecules on the basis of their density and shape using the gravitational field generated in a high-speed centrifuge. It is used in rDNA work for the separation of RNA and DNA, and for purification of plasmids.

Ultrafiltration

Molecular sieves; membranes with pores small enough to remove large molecules. Rated in terms of nominal molecular weight cutoff. A 10,000 Dalton (molecular weight) UF membrane, for example, will remove bacterial pyrogens that are typically in the range of 20,000 Daltons.

Ultrafine Particle

Particle with an equivalent diameter less than 0,1μm.

Ultrapure Water

Water with a specific resistance higher than 1 megohm-cm. In the laboratory, it usually refers to Type I reagent grade water.

Anything in laboratory water that is not H2O is an impurity. Although chemically pure water is not attainable, ultrapure water systems are now capable of reducing impurities down to the limits of detection.

Ultraviolet Oxidation

Ultraviolet radiation is employed in water purification for the photochemical oxidation of organic impurities resulting in HPLC grade water with organic impurity levels below 0.0005 absorbance units.

Ultraviolet Radiation

Light in the wavelength region 200-300 nm, used to detect RNA or DNA that has the fluorescent dye, ethidium bromide, bound to it.

Ultraviolet Sterilizer

Ultraviolet lamps used to kill microorganisms in water.

Ultraviolet TOC Reduction

An ultraviolet source, which partially oxidizes organic compounds to ionic species that can be removed. It relies on 185 nm (nanometer) radiation from "ozone producing" mercury lamps (along with 254nm germicidal radiation). Generally has a longer contact time than sterilization alone.

Unicellular

Composed of only a single cell.

Unidirectional Airflow

Previously referred as "laminar" airflow, is the "rectified airflow through the entire cross section of a clean zone with a steady velocity and approximately parallel streamlines. This type of airflow results in a directed transport of particles from the clean zone".

Uniform Building Code (UBC)

The most widely adopted model building code in the United States is a performance based document meeting the needs of government units charged with the enforcement of building regulations.

Uniform Fire Code™

The premier model fire code in the United States sets forth provisions necessary for fire prevention and fire protection. Published by the International Fire Code Institute (IFCI) and endorsed by the Western Fire Chiefs Association, the International Association of Fire Chiefs, and the International Conference of Building Officials (ICBO), it contains code provisions compatible with the Uniform Building Code, and standards referenced from the code provisions.

Uniform Mechanical Code™

A document that provides a complete set of requirements for the design, construction, installation, and maintenance of heating, ventilating, cooling and refrigeration systems; incinerators and other heat-producing appliances.

Uniform Zoning Code™

A code dedicated to intelligent community development and to the benefit of the public welfare by providing a means of promoting uniformity in zoning laws and enforcement.

Unit Dose Defines an SVP that must be administered in one dose. Universal Precautions

Precautions taken when handling, storing, transporting, or shipping items or specimens containing, or contaminated with human blood and body fluids: all such materials are treated as infectious.

Unsaturated Fatty Acid

A fatty acid containing one or more double bonds.

Usnea (Usnea barbata)

Antimicrobial.

Unstable

An unstable compound is one which will spontaneously

decompose or transform into other compounds over a relatively short period of time.

Unstable (Reactive) Material

A material other than an explosive, which in the pure state or as commercially produced will vigorously polymerize, decompose, condense or become self-reactive and undergo other violent chemical changes, including explosion, when exposed to heat, friction or shock, or in the absence of an inhibitor or in the presence of contaminants or in contact with noncompatible materials. Unstable, reactive materials are subdivided as follows:

1. Class 4 - Materials that in themselves are readily capable of detonation or of explosive decomposition or explosive reaction at normal temperatures and pressures. This class includes materials that are sensitive to mechanical or localized thermal shock at normal temperatures and pressures.
2. Class 3 - Materials that in themselves, are capable of detonation or of explosive decomposition or explosive reaction but which require a strong initiating source or which must be heated under confinement before initiation. This class includes materials that are sensitive to thermal or mechanical shock at elevated temperatures and pressures.
3. Class 2 - Materials that in themselves are normally unstable and readily undergo violent chemical change but do not detonate. This class includes materials which can undergo chemical change with rapid release of energy at normal temperatures and pressures and which can undergo violent chemical change at elevated temperatures and pressures.
4. Class 1 - Materials that in themselves are normally stable but which can become unstable at elevated temperatures and pressures.

Upward Compatibility

Refers to software that runs not only on the computer for which it was designed, but also on newer and more powerful models. In the context of CFR 21 Part 11, compatibility plays an important role in ensuring that legacy data can be moved (copied) accurately and completely to a new system. Without it, legacy systems would have to be maintained as long as the records contained in them are kept.

Uracil

A pyrimidine base important as a component of ribonucleic acid (RNA). Uracil is capable of forming a base pair with adenine.

User Interface

Dials, knobs, operating system commands, graphical display formats, and other devices provided by a computer or a program to allow users to communicate and use the computer or program. A Graphical User Interface (GUI) provides its user with a "picture oriented" way to interact with technology.

U.S.P. (United States Pharmacopeia)

A compendium of testing and purity criteria for pharmaceuticals, ancillaries, and raw materials. (also see: National Formulary (NF))

Utility Systems

Facility wide systems not tailored to a specific process and that do not have contact with the drug substance or potential drug substance.

V

Vacuoles

Membrane-bound organelles of low density responsible for food digestion, osmotic regulation, and waste product storage. Vacuoles may occupy a large fraction of cell volume (up to 90% in plant cells).

Vaccine

A preparation of microbial antigens that provokes an immune response (i.e. the production of antibodies) on injection, thus conferring immunity on the recipient. There are three types of vaccines:

1. Those containing material from a nonvirulent organism that retains its immunogenicity but does not result in infection.
2. Those containing a modified toxin (a toxoid) that has lost its toxic properties but retain its immunogenicity.
3. Those containing live, attenuated organisms (i.e. genetic variants of a virus or bacterium) that are antigenically similar to the original strain but lack virulence.

Recombinant DNA research has allowed the production of new and more specific vaccines. For example, the gene for the B antigen of hepatitis virus has been cloned in E. coli, the protein expressed and a specific anti-B antiserum produced which can be used as a vaccine.

A preparation of killed microorganisms, living attenuated organisms, or living fully virulent organisms that is administered to produce or artificially increase immunity to a particular disease.

Vacuum Degasification

The process of removing dissolved and entrained gases from the Reverse Osmosis (RO) product water by creating a vacuum in a tower through which this water flows. The degasifier may be located before the RO system but the majority of the time will be located after. The most prevalent gas present is Carbon Dioxide (CO2), which may have been generated during pH adjustment of the RO feed water. The anion exchange resin can remove CO2 but using the vacuum degasifier can reduce that load. The other gas of concern is Oxygen, which can also be removed by a vacuum degasifier.

Valerian Root (Valeriana officinalis)

Reduces stress; induces sleep76; (European studies show that the major component, the "valepotriates" have sedative, anti-convulsive, hypotensive, tranquilizing, and anti-aggressive qualities, making Valerian a natural tranquilizer77.)

Validation

A documented program that provides a high degree of assurance that a specific process, method, or system will consistently produce a result meeting pre-determined acceptance criteria.

Validation Master Plan

The documented plan for qualification of a facility or part of a facility that identifies the layout of the operation, the associated utilities and systems, the equipment, and the processes to be validated. The validation master plan also provides preliminary information as to the extent of the qualification and validation (IQ, OQ, PQ), required documentation, SOPs, acceptance criteria and responsibilities. Validation Master Plans should also establish the cross reference of qualification projects by product, system, discipline, etc.

Validation Protocol

A written plan describing the process to be validated, including production equipment and how validation will be conducted. Such a plan would address objective test parameters, product and process characteristics, predetermined specifications, and factors, which will determine acceptable results.

Validation Protocol (from ICH API)

A written plan stating how validation will be conducted and defining acceptance criteria. For example, the protocol for a manufacturing process identifies processing equipment, critical process parameters/operating ranges, product characteristics, sampling, and test data to be collected, number of validation runs, and acceptable test results.

Vanilla

Vanilla is a flavouring, in its pure form known as vanillin, derived from orchids in the genus Vanilla. The name came from the Spanish word "vainilla", diminutive form of "vaina" (meaning "sheath"), which is in turn derived from Latin "vagina".

Vanilla is a flavouring essence prepared from the seed-pods of Vanilla orchids. The species harvested for vanillin (there are in fact several) is mainly Vanilla planifolia. It is a native of Mexico, though now widely grown throughout the tropics. Madagascar is one of the largest producers. Additional sources include Vanilla pompona and Vanilla tahitiensis.

Though there are many compounds present in the extracts of vanilla, the compound predominantly responsible for the characteristic flavour and smell of vanilla is known as vanillin. Vanilla essence comes in two forms: the actual extract of the seedpods, and the far cheaper synthetic essence, basically consisting of a solution of synthetic vanillin (4-hydroxy-3-methoxybenzaldehyde):

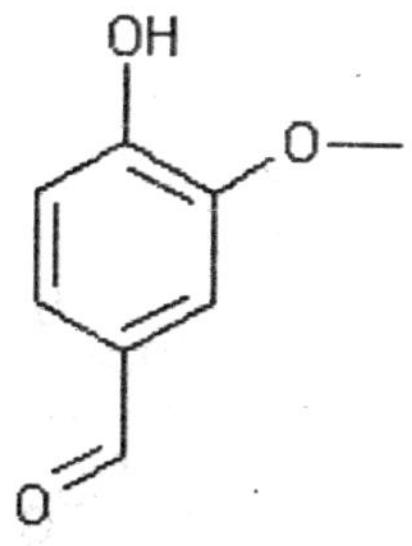

Vanillin
(4-hydroxy-3-methoxybenzaldehyde)

Natural vanilla is an extremely complicated mixture of several hundred different compounds, versus synthetic vanillin which is derived from phenol and is of high purity. However, it may be difficult to determine the difference between natural and synthetic vanilla flavouring.

Vanilla flavour in creams, cakes and other foodstuff may be achieved by adding some vanilla essence or by cooking vanilla beans in the liquid preparation. A stronger aroma may be attained if the beans are split in two; in this case, the innards of the beans, consisting of flavourful tiny black grains, are mixed into the preparation.

Good quality vanilla has a strong aromatic flavour, but foodstuffs with small amounts of low quality vanilla or artificial vanilla-like flavourings are far more common, since true vanilla is much more expensive.

One major use of vanilla is in flavouring ice cream: the most common flavour of ice cream is vanilla, and thus most people consider it to be the "default" flavour.

By analogy, the term "plain vanilla" or just "vanilla" is used for default i.e. with no extras or modifications, in many situations, for example vanilla sex. Since "plain vanilla" ice creams often do not have a strong vanilla taste, the term "French vanilla" is often used to designate preparations that actually have a strong vanilla aroma, and possibly contain vanilla grains.

Vanilla was a well regarded flavouring in Pre-Columbian Mesoamerica, and was brought back to Europe (and from there the rest of the world) by the Spanish Conquistadors.

In ancient Mexico the Totonac people were regarded as the producers of the best vanilla. They continued to be the world's chief producers of the flavouring through the mid 19th century. At that time, French Vanilla *growers in Mexico traded their knowledge of artificial pollination of flowers for the Totonac knowledge of preparing the beans.*

Some connoisseurs still regard the Totonac vanilla as the best. Such is sometimes marketed in gourmet food stores as "Mexican vanilla", although Mexico also produces low quality vanilla that sometimes shares this label.

The Coca-Cola Corporation is the world's largest customer of natural vanilla extract. When New Coke was introduced in 1985, the economy of Madagascar crashed, and only recovered after New Coke flopped. The reason was that New Coke uses vanillin, a less-expensive synthetic substitute, and purchases of vanilla more than halved during this period. By 2002, the company introduced Vanilla Coke which is Coca-Cola with vanilla flavour.

Vapor Pressure

Dalton's Law for a mixture of perfect gases states that the mixture pressure is equal to the sum of the partial pressures of the constituents. The partial pressure of moisture is called vapor pressure, and is expressed as: Total Pressure (Pt) = Partial Pressure of Air (Pa) + Partial Pressure of Moisture (Pv).

Vasaka

The drug consists of the leaves of *Adhatoda vasica* Nees.

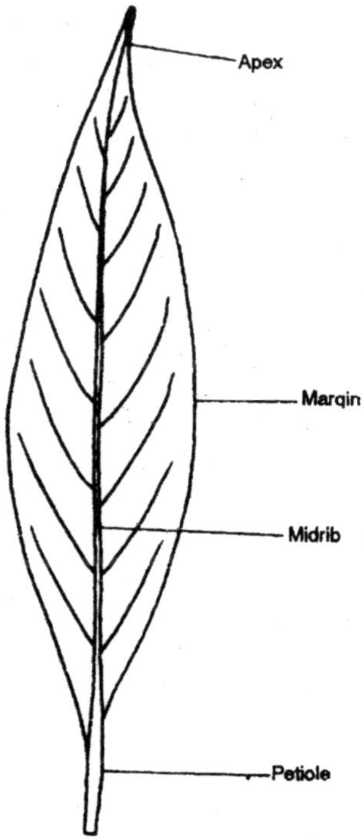

Vasaka Leaf

Vascular Targeting Agents (VTAs)

Multifunctional agents that are home to the capillaries and vessels of solid tumors.

Vector

An agent, such as an insect, that can carry a disease-producing organism from one host to another; the agent used to carry new genes into cells. Plasmids currently are the vectors of choice, though viruses and other bacteria may sometimes be used. These molecules become part of the cell protoplasm.

VEAs (Vasopermeation Enhancement Agents)

A new generation of drugs that increase the uptake of therapeutic agents to solid tumors.

Vegetative

Form In bacteria, a stage of active growth, as opposed to a resting state or spore formation.

Vehicle

Any solvent or carrier fluid in a pharmaceutical product that has no pharmacological role. For example, water is the vehicle for xilocaine and propylene glycol is the vehicle for many antibiotics.

Verification

The act of reviewing, inspecting, testing, checking, auditing, or otherwise establishing and documenting whether items, processes, services, or documents conform to specified requirements. (also see: IQ (Installation Qualification))

Veterinary

Referring to pharmaceuticals or biologicals intended for animal use. Historically veterinary products were made by less than "Good Manufacturing Products". Today, however, the GMP's refer to both human and veterinary products.

Viable Living

Viable Organism Capable of living and reproducing. Thus,

nothing is sterile as long as it contains even a single viable organism.

Vial

A final container for a parenteral or diagnostic product. Sealed with a rubber closure and over-seal. Generally required to be class I borosilicate glass.

Vinca

Vinca is the dried whoe plant of *Catharanthus roseus* G. Don.

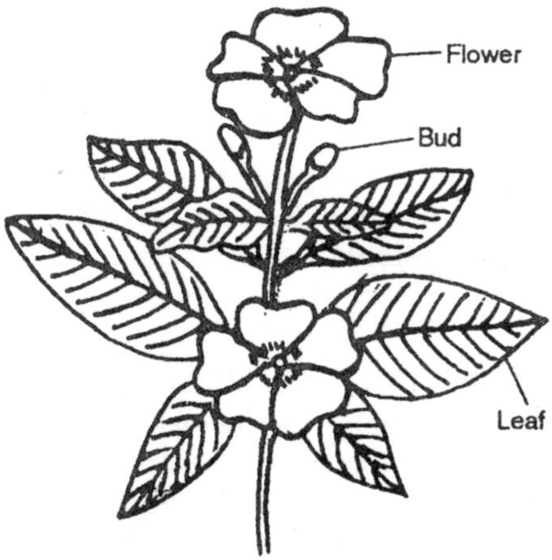

Vinca plant

Viral Antigens

Specific proteins on the capsid of a virus that can act as inducers of antibody formation.

Virion

A fully formed, mature virus. Infection is initiated in a cell by a virion.

Virucide

An agent that destroys or inactivates viruses.

Virulence

The disease-producing power of a microorganism.

Virus

A simple, noncellular parasite that can reproduce only inside living cells. The simple structure of viruses is their most important characteristic. Most of them consist only of a genetic material - either DNA or RNA - and a protein coating. Some also have membranous envelopes. Viruses are "alive" in that they can reproduce themselves - although only by taking over a cell's synthetic machinery - but they have none of the other characteristics of living organisms. Viruses cause a large variety of significant diseases in plants and animals, including humans.

Viscosity

The tendency of a fluid to resist flowing because of molecular attraction (cohesion).

Vitamin

Term coined in 1911 (vita, Latin word for life, and the chemical term amine) by polish biochemist, Casimir Funk, represents one of a group of organic substances, some of which are of unknown composition, present in minute amount in natural foodstuffs which are essential to normal metabolism. A lack of which in the dietary causes deficiency diseases. Vitamins are commonly classified into two groups, the fat-soluble, and the water-soluble. Vitamins A, D, E, and K are fat-soluble. Vitamin C and members of the vitamin B complex group are water-soluble. In general, the vitamins play catalytic and regulatory roles in the body's metabolism. Among the water-soluble vitamins, the B vitamins apparently function as coenzymes. Vitamin's C coenzyme role, if any, has not been established. Part of the importance of vitamin C to the body may result from its strong antioxidant action. The actions of the fat-soluble vitamins are less well understood. Some of them, too, may contribute to enzyme activity, and some of them are essential to the functioning of cellular membranes.

Volatile

A substance which evaporates easily is said to be 'volatile.' Things with a strong aroma are generally volatile, because the molecules easily pass into the surrounding air.

Volatile or Essential Oils

Volatile oils are usually responsible for the odor of a plant. Volatile, or essential, oils evaporate with air. They can contain hundreds of constituents, the highest of which are terpenes. Hydrocarbons (as with acillin, from garlic), alcohols, aldehydes (this group includes cinnamon oil, orange oil, lemon peel, lemon oil, hamamelis water, and citronella oil, whose medicinal purposes include the astringent quality of witch hazel). Therapeutically, volatile oils have many uses. They can serve as a mode of transportation, to distribute a medicine equally throughout the body. They can act as antiseptics. Volatile oils tend to stimulate tissues they come in contact with, hence they can be rubefacients, counter-irritants, and/or vasodilators. Internally, volatile oils may cause an increase in saliva, perspiration, peristalsis, and/or stimulate the heart muscle.

Volatile oils

Generic name for a heterogeneous class of low-boiling, usually fat-soluble, low molecular weight plant constituents which includes low molecular weight terpenes, polypeptides, and aliphatic compounds; syn: essential oils.

Voltage-dependent calcium and sodium ion channels

Ion channels are pores in the cell membrane, especially in nerve cells, that allow the passage of ions (an electrically charged atom or molecule) in and out of cells. Ion channels play an important role in the maintenance of electrical charge differential between inside and outside of the cell membrane. The opening and closing of the voltage-dependent ion channels is regulated by voltage, which is the electrical charge or potential difference between the inside and outside of the membrane.

VPHP

Microbiodecontamination Technology used to decontaminate

the exposed, internal surfaces within a sealed isolator and the exposed, external surfaces of materials and components placed within the sealed isolator. It consists of four distinctive phases: 1. Dehumidification - Lowers humidity and increases temperature 2. Conditioning - "Ramp-up" (VPHP) at or below saturation conditions 3. Sterilization - Steady-State (VPHP) at or below saturation conditions 4. Aeration - Reduces the VPHP to Safe Levels.

W

WAN(Wide Area Network)

Network with computers far apart, connected by telephone lines or radio waves.LAN (Local Area Network))

Warning Letter

The most serious FDA postaudit (after inspection) letter notifying a manufacturer of adverse finding and giving it 15 days to reply.

Wasabi

Wasabi (Japanese: □□ or □□□; scientific name Wasabia japonica (syn. Cochlearia wasabi, Eutrema japonica)) is a member of the cabbage family. Commonly known as Japanese horseradish, it grows naturally along stream beds in mountain river valleys in Japan. There are also other species used such as W. koreana, and W. tetsuigi. The two main cultivars in the marketplace are W. japonica var. Duruma and Mazuma. There are many others though. It is green and has an extremely strong flavor. Its hotness is different from that of chile peppers, which burn the tongue; wasabi produces *vapors that burn* the sinus cavity instead.

It is sold either in root form, which must be finely grated before use, or as a dried powder which is then mixed with water to make a paste. In both cases, the hot taste develops after a few minutes; both the ungrated root and the dry powder taste rather dull. It is also sold as a ready-to-use paste, which comes in tubes approximately the size and shape of travel toothpaste tubes. Once the paste is prepared you should cover it until served to protect the flavor.

Fresh leaves of wasabi can also be eaten and have some of wasabi root's hot flavor. They can be eaten as wasabi salad by pickling overnight with a salt and vinegar based dressing, or by quickly boiling them with a little soy sauce. Additionally, the leaves are battered and deep-fried into chips.

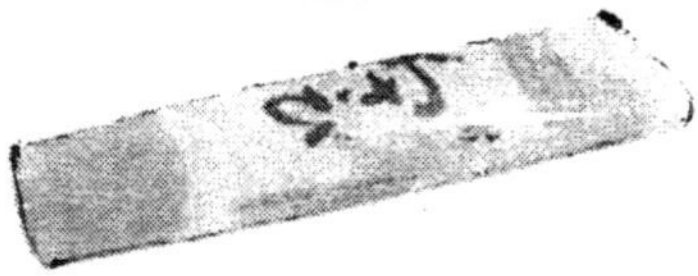

A tube of wasabi

Fortunately for those who either through malice or unfamiliarity come into contact with too much of this condiment, the burning sensations it can induce are short-lived compared to the effects of chile peppers. When used as intended, it is also very tasty on roasted peas, or in small amounts on sushi or sashimi. Wasabi is commonly mixed with soy sauce to make a dipping sauce for sushi and sashimi. However, wasabi's flavor dissolves very quickly in water and the best way to enjoy wasabi is to apply wasabi after dipping into soy sauce or carefully avoiding wasabi from mixing with soy sauce.

Washout period

Period required for a substance or medication to be cleared completely from the body.

Water Hammer

A tremendous force produced by rapid interruption of linear flow of a non-compressible fluid. Most commonly occurs when fast acting valves are closed in a high flow liquid system.

Water Treatment

Water treatment, also referred to as water conditioning, can consist of adding or removing chemicals to change the properties of water. In water softening, for example, sodium ions are substituted for metallic ions that cause "hardness" thus reducing the scale-forming tendencies of water. Water purification on the other hand, always consists of removing undesirable impurities.

Waviness

The more widely spaced component of surface texture. Unless otherwise noted, waviness includes all irregularities whose spacing is greater than the roughness sampling length. Waviness may result from such factors as machine or work deflection, vibration, chatter, heat treatment or warping strains. Roughness may be considered as superimposed on a "wavy" surface.

Western Blot

A procedure in which a mixture of proteins is separated on a polyacrylamide gel and then transferred to a nylon membrane. The membrane may then be treated with reagents such as specific antibodies to locate a protein of interest.

Wetted Surface

The surface(s) of any valve or component that will be exposed to a fluid (liquid or gas) when in service.

WFI (Water For injection), U.S.P.

WFI is water purified by distillation or by reverse osmosis, it contains no added substance. WFI meets the purity requirements under Purified Water. Although not intended to be sterile, it meets a test for a limit of bacterial endotoxin. It must be produced, stored, and distributed under Sterile Water for Injection.

White Blood Cell

A blood cell containing no respiratory pigment. In vertebrates it may be a polymorphonuclear leukocyte, a lymphocyte or a monocyte.

White oak bark (Quercus alba)

Anti-inflammatory; helps prevent diarrhea.

White pine bark (Pinus strobus)
Expectorant.

White willow (Salix alba)
pain reliever78; relieves headaches, fevers, arthritis, sore muscles, and chills79.

White cherry bark (Prunus serotina)
Respiratory

Wild yam (Dioscorea villosa)
Increases liver efficiency by lowering serum cholesterol80; helps prevent miscarriage;reduces dysmenorrhea, cramps, and afterpain (uterine cramps after giving birth)81.

Wild cherry bark (Prunus serotina)
Astringent; helps irritating coughs due to sedative action, anti-tussive, expectorant, Note that inhibition of a cough does not chest infection, which will still need to be treated.

Wintergreen (Gaultheria procumbens)
Anodyne; astringent; diuretic; stimulant; emmenagoge; lactagogue.

Workstation
An open or enclosed work surface, usually with direct air supply.

Worst Case
The highest or lowest value of a given control parameter actually evaluated in a validation exercise.

Wool
Wool consists of more or less curved, subcylindrical threads, covered with irregular lines crossing them transversely at fairly close intervals and connected by other lines at right angles to them. A dark coloured narrow band is present along the central axis of many of the hairs and is called medulla. The fibres are about 15 to 25 or 45 to 60 μ in width. Wool fibre

polarise brightly with crossed nicols, many hair show bright colour.

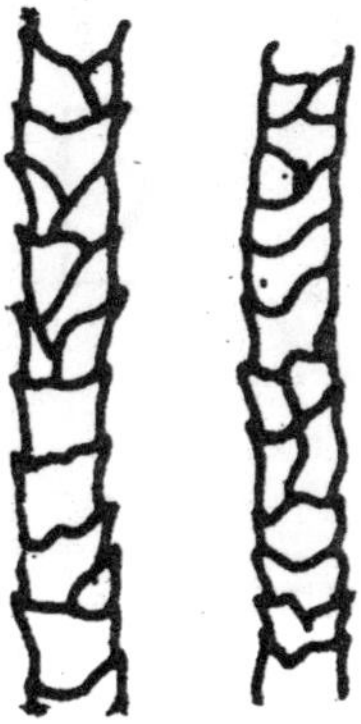

Wool fibre

X

X Chromosome

A sex chromosome that usually occurs paired in each female cell and single in each male cell in species in which the male typically has two unlike cell chromosomes.

Xenobiotics

Industrial chemicals that have a chemical structure not found in natural compounds that may resist degradation by microorganisms.

XPS(X-Ray Photoelectron Spectroscopy) or ESCA (Electron Spectroscopy for Chemical Analysis)

A surface-sensitive technique capable of detecting all elements with an atomic number greater than that of helium. ESCA provides data on the outermost several atomic layers of a material, and has a sensitivity in the order of 0.5 atomic percent. A primary advantage of ESCA is that it can both determine and quantify the chemical state of the elements detected (i.e. metallic state or oxide state).

Y

Y Chromosome

A sex chromosome that is characteristic of male zygotes in species in which the male typically has two unlike sex chromosomes.

Yarrow (Achillea millefolium)

Purifies the blood; reduces fever; lowers blood pressure; digestive stimulant; diaphoretic.

Yeast Artificial Chromosome

A vector used to clone DNA fragments (up to 400 kb); it is constructed from the telomeric, centromeric, and replication origin sequences needed for replication in yeast cells.

Yeasts

Unicellular fungi belonging mainly to the Ascomycetes that usually multiply by budding. Their commercial significance lies in their ability to secrete enzymes. For example, in the brewing and baking industries, it is a source of vitamins and proteins. They can also be used as excipients in rDNA technology.

Yellow Dock (Rumex crispus)

Clears skin problems including eczema and psoriasis; relieves glandular inflammation and swelling; eliminates ringworm;

In India yellow Dock even hardened weak gums (softened by having a bad diet82); also has some antibiotic properties83.

Yerba Santa (Eriodictyon californicum)

Respiratory.

Yield, Expected

The quantity of material or the percentage of theoretical yield anticipated at any appropriate phase of production based on previous laboratory, pilot scale, or manufacturing data.

Yield, Theoretical

The quantity that would be produced at any appropriate phase of manufacture, processing, or packing of a particular API (Active Pharmaceutical Ingredient) or intermediate, based upon the quantity of components to be used, in the absence of any loss or error in actual production.

Yucca Root (Yucca species)

Anti-inflammatory for arthritis.

Z

Za'atar

Za'atar (sometimes spelled **Zaatar** or **Zatar**) is a popular mixture of spices that originated in the Middle East. It is traditionally composed of marjoram, wild oregano, thyme, toasted white sesame seeds, and sumac. Some sources list savory and salt as well as fennel. Different versions of za'atar will differ greatly in the proportion of each spice included. In Lebanon there is a belief that this particular spice mixture makes the mind alert and the body strong. For this reason, children are encouraged to eat a za'atar sandwich for breakfast before an exam. The mixture is also popular in Turkey, Syria, Jordan, Israel, and North Africa. It is used to spice meats and vegetables, and it is also mixed with olive oil to make a spread (za'atar-ul-zayt or zayt-tu-zaa'tar), used as a dip for sesame rings (kay-ak). Za'atar can also be spread on little bread rolls, the equivalent of a mini pizza.

Zedoary

Zedoary *(Curcuma zedoaria)* is the name for a perennial herb and member of the ginger family (Zingiberaceae). The plant is native to India and Indonesia. It was introduced to Europe by Arabs around the sixth century, but its use as a spice in the West today is extremely *rare, having been replaced by ginger.* Zedoary is a rhizome that grows in tropical and subtropical wet forest regions. The fragrant plant bears yellow flowers with red and green bracts and the underground stem section is large and tuberous with numerous branches. The leaf shoots of the zedoary are long and can reach 1 metre (3 feet) in height.

The edible root of zedoary has a bright orange interior and a fragrance reminiscent of mango, however its flavour is more similar to ginger, except with a very bitter aftertaste. In Indonesia it is ground to a powder and added to curry pastes, whereas in India it tends to be used fresh or pickled.

Zedoary is also used in some traditional eastern medicines where it is reputed to be an aid to digestion, a relief for colic and an agent for purifying the blood.

Zeolite

Naturally occurring or synthetic permutite, a hydrated alkali-aluminum silicate that exhibits limited base exchange. Used as an ion exchange medium for the softening of hard water.

Zeta Potential

The charge or potential existing at the surface of a particle. It is the positive charge measured at the surface of the membrane across the pH range.

Zoonosis

Any disease in humans acquired from one of the lower animals, rabies is an example.

Zygote

Single cell formed from the conjugation of gametes (egg and sperm cells). The zygote has twice as many chromosomes as do gametes.